Atlas of Clear Cell Carcinoma of the Ovary

Junzo Kigawa • Tsunehisa Kaku • Toru Sugiyama
Steven G. Silverberg

Atlas of Clear Cell Carcinoma of the Ovary

A Pathological Guide

Springer

Junzo Kigawa
Matsue City Hospital
Matsue
Shimane
Japan

Tsunehisa Kaku
Department of Health Sciences
Department of Health Sciences Graduate School of Medical Sciences
Fukuoka
Fukuoka
Japan

Toru Sugiyama
Department of Obstetrics and Gynecology
Iwate Medical University School of Medicine
Morioka
Iwate
Japan

Steven G. Silverberg
Department of Pathology,
University of Maryland School of Medicine
Baltimore, MD
USA

ISBN 978-4-431-55437-0 ISBN 978-4-431-55438-7 (eBook)
DOI 10.1007/978-4-431-55438-7

Library of Congress Control Number: 2015936039

Springer Tokyo Heidelberg New York Dordrecht London

Printed on acid-free paper

Springer Japan KK is part of Springer Science+Business Media (www.springer.com)

Preface

Clear cell carcinoma of the ovary (CCC) was originally termed "mesonephroid" by Schiller in 1939 as it was thought to originate from mesonephric structures and resembled renal carcinoma [1]. Since 1973, CCC has been recognized as a distinct histologic entity in the World Health Organization (WHO) classification of ovarian tumors [2]. CCC is characterized by clear epithelial cells containing abundant cytoplasmic glycogen and hobnail cells, either alone or in combination. Tumors are diagnosed as CCC if the following are recognized: a small to large sheet of polyhedral clear cells with delicate fibrovascular septa; tubules and papillae; clear, hobnail, or eosinophilic cells of organoid appearance; or clear cells with coalescent vacuoles containing "targetoid" eosinophilic PAS-positive globules.

Recently, the Japanese Gynecologic Oncology Group (JGOG) and the Gynecologic Cancer Intergroup (GCIG) conducted a clinical trial for CCC (JGOG3017), and 652 cases were collected and a central pathological review was performed using a virtual slide system (NanoZommer C9600, Hamamatsu Photonics KK). In this trial, an international central pathological review (CPR) was done by 21 expert gynecologic pathologists from six countries. Cases with disagreement on the diagnosis of CCC were discussed in an international teleconference system (3e C Conference system by Kimura Information Technology). The disagreement rate was 3.1 %.

Several interesting and important histological features of CCC were noted in the process of CPR such as growth patterns (papillary, tubocystic, solid and adenofibromatous), cell types (classical hobnail and clear cell, eosinophilic, and oxyphilic), stromal changes (hyalinized, necrotic, hemorrhagic, lymphocytic infiltrative, luteinized, and psammomatous calcification), presence of endometriosis and atypical endometriosis, and borderline clear cell tumors. Finally, differential diagnosis is also very important. Among ovarian epithelial tumors, endometrioid carcinoma with secretory change, mucinous carcinoma, serous carcinoma, and borderline clear cell or serous tumor should be excluded. Among germ cell and stromal tumors, yolk sac carcinoma, dysgerminoma, struma ovarii, and steroid cell tumor are also important as differential diagnoses. Metastatic carcinoma should be ruled out. It is very important to understand the typical and unusual histological features of CCC and related tumors for diagnosis and treatment.

We have appreciated the opportunity to review this large series of CCC. Therefore, we are sharing our observations in this atlas of pathology of clear cell carcinoma of the ovary.

Matsue, Shimane, Japan	Junzo Kigawa
Fukuoka, Fukuoka, Japan	Tsunehisa Kaku
Morioka, Iwate, Japan	Toru Sugiyama
Baltimore, MD, USA	Steven G. Silverberg

References

1. Schiller W (1939) Mesonephroma ovarii. Am J Cancer 35:1
2. Serov SF, Scully RE, Sobin LH (1973) International histologic classification of tumors. No.9. Histologic typing of ovarian tumors. World Health Organization, Geneva, p 37

Acknowledgments

We are grateful to the members of the Japanese Gynecologic Oncology Group (JGOG) and the Coordinating Center of Kitasato University.

We specially thank the members of international central pathologic review as follows; Prof. Shinj Fukunaga Jikei University, Dr. Norioko Kato, Hirosaki University, Dr. Shinichi Teshima, The Fraternity Memorial Hospital, Prof. Takako Kiyokawa, Jikei University, Prof. Yoshiki Mikami, Kumamoto University, Dr. Suzuko Moritani, Nagoya Medical Center, Prof. Takuya Moriya, Kawasaki Medical School, Prof. Teiichi Motoyama, Yamagata University, Prof. Tetsuro Nagasaka, Nagoya University, Dr. Yoshihiro Ohishi, Kyushu University, Prof. Hiroyuki Yanai, Okayama University, Prof. Masami Yasuda, Saitama International Medical Center, Dr. Yuko Sasajima, Teikyo University, Dr. Norihiro Teramoto, Shikoku Cancer Center, Prof. Hitoshi Tsuda, National Defence Medical College, Prof. David Millan, Glasgow Royal Infirmary, UK; Prof. In-Sun Kim, Korea University Medical College, Korea; Prof. Simona Losito, National Cancer Institute, Italy, and Prof. Marie Cécile Vacher-Lavenu, Hôpital Cochin, France.

We also thank Dr. Eizo Kimura, Kousei Hospital and Dr. Toyomi Sato, Tukuba University for offering specimens; Dr. Hiroaki Itamochi, Dr. Tetsuro Oishi, Dr. Muneaki Shimada, Dr. Shinya Sato, Tottori University and Dr. Manabu Yoshida, Matsue City Hospital for providing technical support.

Contents

1 Introduction

The incidence of ovarian cancer in 2012 was projected to be 230,000 new cases and 151,905 deaths worldwide, representing 4.3 % of all female cancers and 4.2 % of all cancer deaths in women [1]. Ovarian cancer is one of the major causes of death from cancer in women. Ovarian cancer is one of the most chemosensitive solid tumors, with objective responses ranging from 60 to 80 % even in patients with advanced stage. However, most tumors ultimately recur and develop resistance to chemotherapy [2, 3]. Recently, the biological characteristics of ovarian cancer have been clarified [4]. It has long been known that ovarian cancers of serous histology appear to be more sensitive to chemotherapy than other histological subtypes [5–7]. Patients with clear cell carcinoma (CCC) of the ovary showed a significantly worse prognosis in a retrospective review of several Gynecologic Oncology Group (GOG) trials [5]. Several studies also showed that patients with CCC had a poor prognosis and the low response of CCC to conventional platinum-based chemotherapy has been associated with poor survival [8–11].

CCC of the ovary has unique clinical and biological features. The incidence of CCC among epithelial ovarian cancers (EOC) differs among races. In North America and Europe, CCC is the third most common histological subtype of EOC, with an estimated prevalence of 1–12 % [12–15]. CCC comprises more than 20 % of such cancers in Japan [16]. Interestingly, among Asian women living in the United States, CCC was diagnosed twice as frequently (11.1 %) compared to Caucasians (4.8 %) [7, 17].

Several studies have analyzed the risk factors for ovarian cancer by histological subtype. CCC was associated (odds ratio 2.3; 95 % confidence interval 1.2–4.2) with an increased body mass index (BMI ≥30) [18]. However, in the NIH-AARP Diet and Health Study, BMI was correlated only with endometrioid histology [19]. It has long been recognized that CCC often is associated with endometriosis (22–70 %), whereas hobnail cells bear a very strong morphological resemblance to endometrial Arias-Stella cells [20, 21]. Endometriosis frequently shows a sequential change to EOC, including CCC. Therefore, atypical endometriosis is considered to be a precancerous change. Ovarian cancers associated with endometriosis tend to occur in younger women and present 5–6 years earlier, on average, than high-grade serous carcinoma. In National Cancer Institute Surveillance, Epidemiology, and End Results (SEER) data, women with CCC were younger than patients with serous adenocarcinoma (SAC) (55 vs. 64 years; median age) [22].

Ovarian CCC usually presents as a large pelvic mass. The size ranges from 3 to 20 cm, with most tumors detected preoperatively either by clinical examination or imaging [12–14, 23]. Recent reports involving large institutional cohorts compared early-stage (I/II) to advanced-stage ovarian cancers (III/IV) and showed that 57–81 % of CCC were diagnosed at an early stage [9–11]; in SEER data, 56 % of CCC was stage I, compared to 19 % for SAC. Combining the low overall incidence of CCC and their early-stage propensity [24], CCC may make up only 1–5 % of advanced-stage patients in chemotherapy trials, largely due to their overall low incidence and tendency for early-stage distribution at the time of initial diagnosis.

Recently, JGOG/GCIG conducted a clinical trial for CCC, and 652 cases were collected and international central pathological review was performed. This study is the largest yet reported. As a result, several interesting and important histological features of CCC were noted in the process of CPR. It is important to understand typical and unusual histological features of CCC and related tumors for diagnosis.

J. Kigawa et al., *Atlas of Clear Cell Carcinoma of the Ovary: A Pathological Guide*,
DOI 10.1007/978-4-431-55438-7_1, © Springer Japan 2015

References

1. International Agency for Research on Cancer. http://globocan.iarc.fr
2. Jemal A, Siegel R, Ward E et al (2007) Cancer statistics. Cancer J Clin 57:43–66
3. Conte PF, Cianci C, Gadducci A (1999) Update in the management of advanced ovarian carcinoma. Crit Rev Oncol Hematol 32:49–58
4. Bast RC Jr, Hennessy B, Mills GB (2009) The biology of ovarian cancer: new opportunities for translation. Nat Rev Cancer 9:415–428
5. Winter WE 3rd, Maxwell GL, Tian C et al (2007) Prognostic factors for stage III epithelial ovarian cancer: a Gynecologic Oncology Group Study. J Clin Oncol 25:3621–3627
6. Ozols RF (2002) Future directions in the treatment of ovarian cancer. Semin Oncol 29:32–42
7. McGuire V, Jesser CA, Whittemore AS (2002) Survival among U.S. women with invasive epithelial ovarian cancer. Gynecol Oncol 84:399–403
8. Gilks CB, Ionescu DN, Kalloger SE et al (2008) Ovarian Cancer Outcomes Unit of the British Columbia Cancer Agency. Tumor cell type can be reproducibly diagnosed and is of independent prognostic significance in patients with maximally debulked ovarian carcinoma. Hum Pathol 39:1239–1251
9. Sugiyama T, Kamura T, Kigawa J et al (2000) Clinical characteristics of clear cell carcinoma of the ovary: a distinct histologic type with poor prognosis and resistance to platinum-based chemotherapy. Cancer 88:2584–2589
10. Takano M, Kikuchi Y, Yaegashi N et al (2006) Clear cell carcinoma of the ovary: a retrospective multicentre experience of 254 patients with complete surgical staging. Br J Cancer 94:1369–1374
11. Itamochi H, Kigawa J, Sugiyama T et al (2002) Low proliferation activity may be associated with chemoresistance in clear cell carcinoma of the ovary. Obstet Gynecol 100:281–287
12. Itamochi H, Kigawa J, Terakawa N (2008) Mechanisms of chemoresistance and poor prognosis in ovarian clear cell carcinoma. Cancer Sci 99:653–658
13. Reed N (2010) Rare and uncommon gynecological cancers, a clinical guide. Springer, Berlin Heidelberg. ISBN:3642134912
14. Kennedy AW, Biscotti CV, Hart WR et al (1989) Ovarian clear cell adenocarcinoma. Gynecol Oncol 32:342–349
15. Crozier MA, Copeland LJ, Silva EG et al (1989) Clear cell carcinoma of the ovary: a study of 59 cases. Gynecol Oncol 35:199–203
16. Japan Society of Obstetrics and Gynecology (2013) Annual report. Acta Obstetrics et Gynecology Japonica 65:1032
17. Jacoby VL, Fujimoto VY, Giudice LC et al (2010) Racial and ethnic disparities in benign gynecologic conditions and associated surgeries. Am J Obstet Gynecol 202:514–521
18. Olsen CM, Nagle CM, Whiteman DC et al (2008) Australian Cancer Study (Ovarian Cancer) and Australian Ovarian Cancer Study Group body size and risk of epithelial ovarian and related cancers: a population-based case-control study. Int J Cancer 123:450–456
19. Pfeiffer RM, Park Y, Kreimer AR et al (2013) Risk prediction for breast, endometrial, and ovarian cancer in white women aged 50 years or older: derivation and validation from population-based cohort studies. PLoS Med 10:e1001492
20. Bulun SE (2009) Endometriosis. N Engl J Med 360:268–279
21. Pearce CL, Templeman C, Rossing MA, Consortium OCA et al (2012) Association between endometriosis and risk of histological subtypes of ovarian cancer: a pooled analysis of case-control studies. Lancet Oncol 13:385–394
22. Mink PJ, Sherman ME, Devesa SS (2002) Incidence patterns of invasive and borderline ovarian tumors among white women and black women in the United States. Results from the SEER Program, 1978–1998. Cancer 95:2380–2389
23. Scarfone G, Bergamini A, Noli S et al (2014) Characteristics of clear cell ovarian cancer arising from endometriosis: a two center cohort study. Gynecol Oncol 133:480–484
24. SEER. http://seer.cancer.gov/csr/1975_2011/results

2 Gross Pathology and Intraoperative Consultation

2.1 Gross Pathology

There is no distinctive gross appearance of ovarian clear cell carcinoma (CCC), which usually is recognizable as malignant but not specifically as CCC. Most of these tumors are solid, soft to firm, and often multinodular, often (especially if large) with foci of necrosis and/or hemorrhage. The color may vary from yellow to white to brown (Fig. 2.1).

A gross finding in some tumors which suggests CCC is one or more foci of tumor within or adjacent to a hemorrhagic smooth-walled cyst with the appearance of endometriosis (Figs. 2.2, 2.3, and 2.4). Most malignant ovarian tumors with this appearance are either CCC or endometrioid adenocarcinoma, with a slight preponderance of the former.

A somewhat different macroscopic appearance is present in those ovarian CCCs of the adenofibromatous type (cf. Chap. 3). Among our cases, 8–9 % expressed this phenotype, of which approximately half were predominantly adenofibromatous. These tumors are usually not obviously grossly malignant and may resemble Brenner tumors or adenofibromas, with a predominantly firm solid architecture punctuated by small or large cystic spaces.

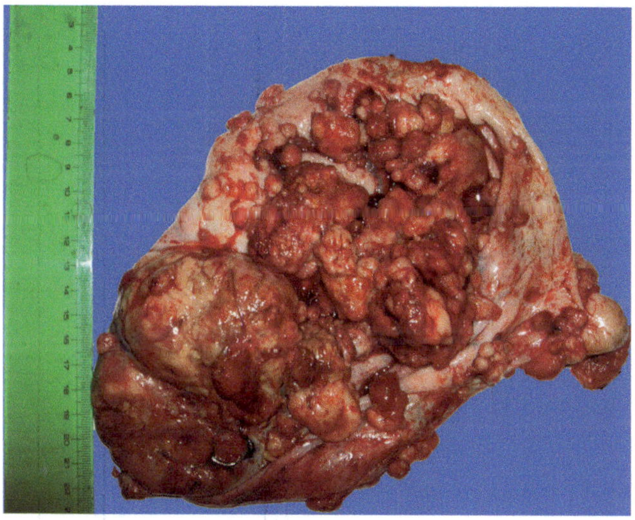

Fig. 2.1 Clear cell carcinoma gross appearance. Large soft multinodular red-gray tumor invading through its capsule. The appearance is malignant but otherwise nonspecific

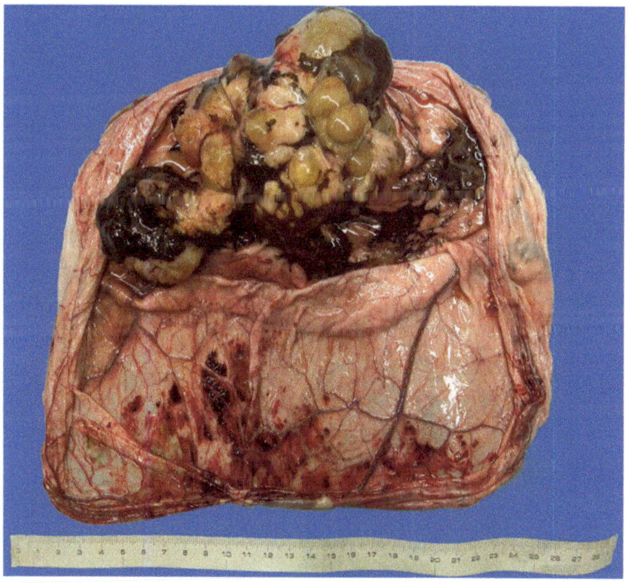

Fig. 2.2 Hemorrhagic smooth-walled endometriotic cyst containing masses of brown necrotic tumor

J. Kigawa et al., *Atlas of Clear Cell Carcinoma of the Ovary: A Pathological Guide*,
DOI 10.1007/978-4-431-55438-7_2, © Springer Japan 2015

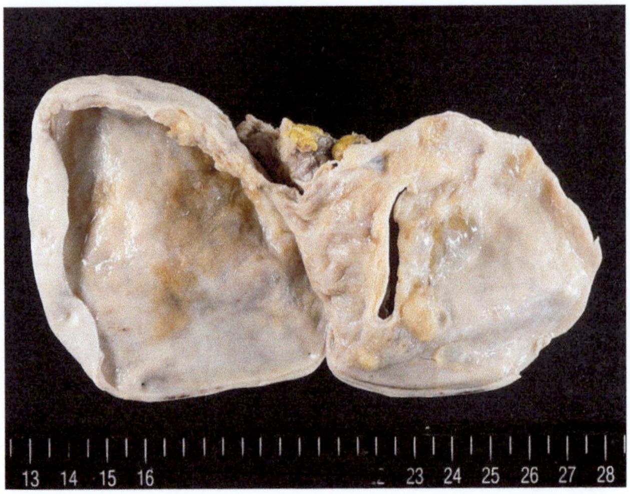

Fig. 2.3 Small solid gray-white tumor foci (R) in cyst lined focally by golden-brown altered blood, representing origin in endometriosis (formalin-fixed specimen)

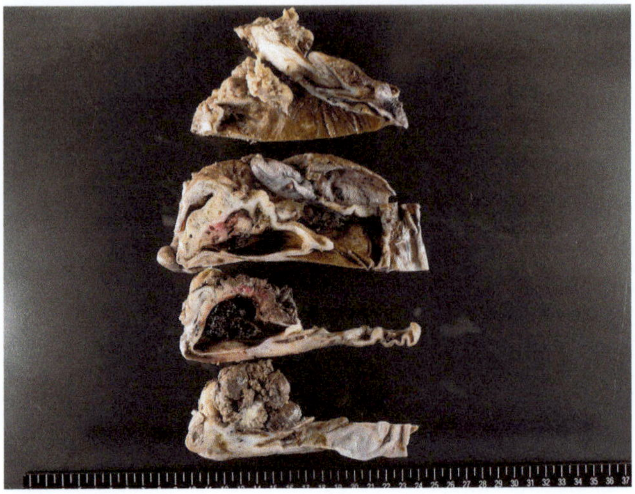

Fig. 2.4 Formalin-fixed and sectioned blood-filled endometriotic cyst surrounded by gray-brown multinodular tumor which is also present in the cyst lumen

2.2 Intraoperative Consultation

2.2.1 Frozen Section

The pathologist is often called for an intraoperative consultation on an ovarian tumor which turns out to be a CCC. As with the gross pathology, in most cases, the diagnosis of adenocarcinoma can be made, but the cell type may be more difficult [1]. Stewart et al. [2] reported that CCC was a more difficult diagnosis by frozen section than was carcinoma of other types, with some CCCs being misclassified as borderline tumors or dysgerminomas.

In cases that we have reviewed, correct diagnosis is directly dependent on frozen section technique. When the slides examined are of only fair quality, architectural crowding and marked nuclear atypia are generally adequate for a malignant diagnosis (Figs. 2.5 and 2.6), but only well-prepared frozen sections from non-necrotic regions of tumor can be diagnosed definitively as CCC (Figs. 2.7, 2.8, and 2.9). As with the gross pathology, frozen sections prepared from CCC regions of adenofibromatous type (Fig. 2.10) may be difficult to classify as malignant.

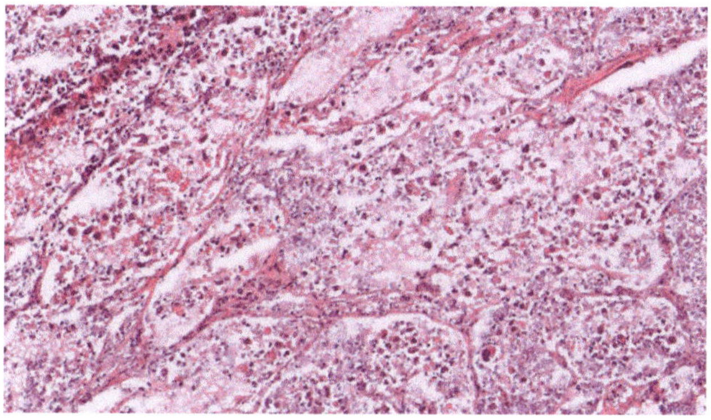

Fig. 2.5 Frozen section of partly necrotic CCC showing tubulocystic architecture with poorly preserved tumor cells

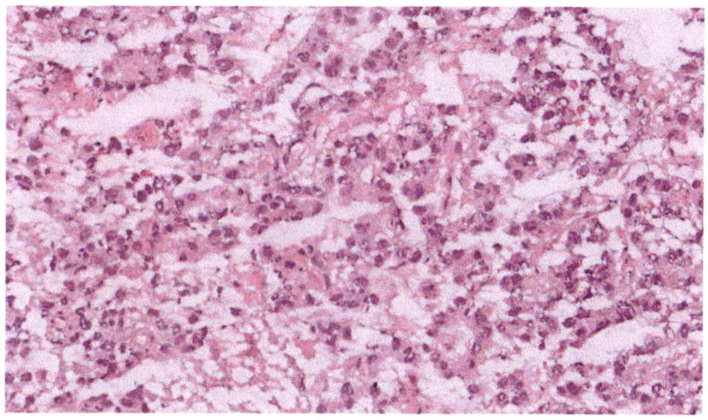

Fig. 2.7 Frozen section from better preserved area in the same tumor, in which malignant clear cells are better visualized

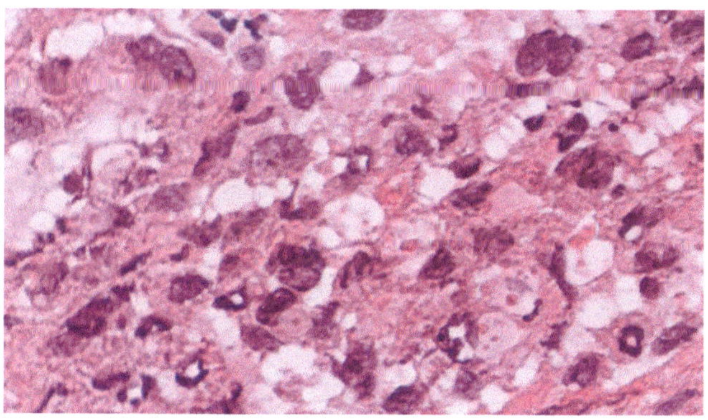

Fig. 2.6 Higher-power magnification of frozen section from a different area of same tumor as Fig. 2.5. Solid nests of markedly atypical tumor cells without mitotic activity or obvious clear cytoplasm

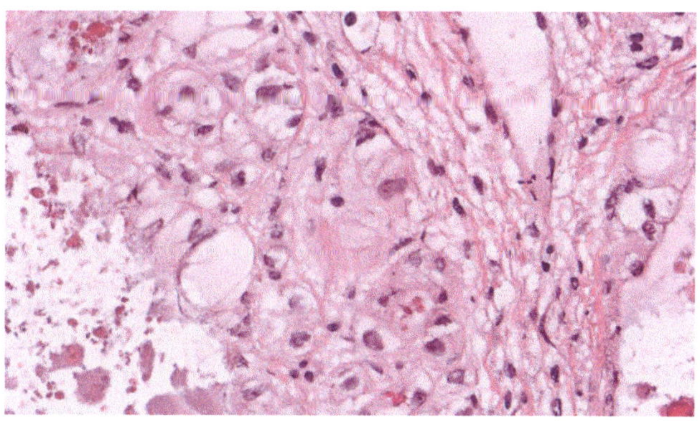

Fig. 2.8 Frozen section of solid focus from a different CCC. Both better tumor preservation and better frozen section technique render malignant clear cells apparent

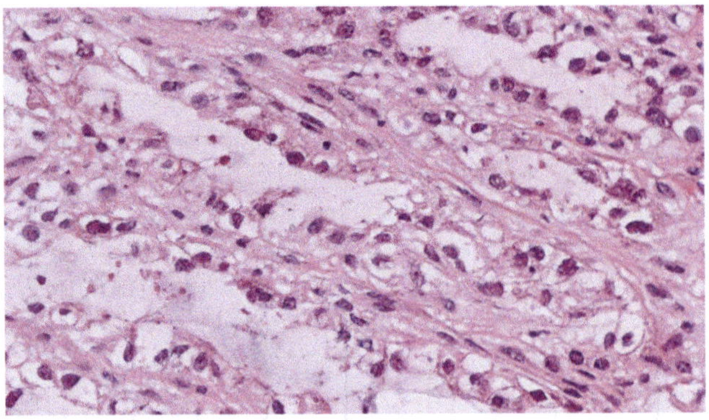

Fig. 2.9 Well-prepared frozen section from well-preserved CCC tubulocystic focus. The diagnosis is easily made from this material

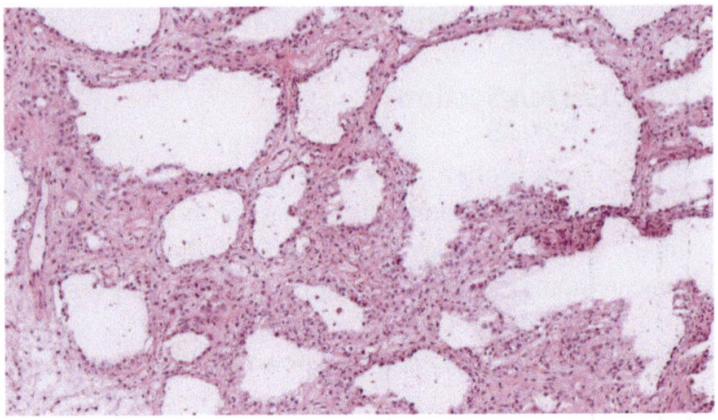

Fig. 2.10 Frozen section of adenofibromatous region of same tumor shown in Figs. 2.8 and 2.9. The diagnosis of both malignancy and cell type depends on the non-adenofibromatous areas

2.2.2 Cytopathology

If intraoperative scrapes or imprints (Figs. 2.11 and 2.12) are prepared from a CCC, both the malignant character and the clear cell morphology may be apparent, especially in air-dried Giemsa-stained preparations (Figs. 2.13 and 2.14). Similar findings are encountered in cytologic preparations from neoplastic ascitic fluid (Fig. 2.15).

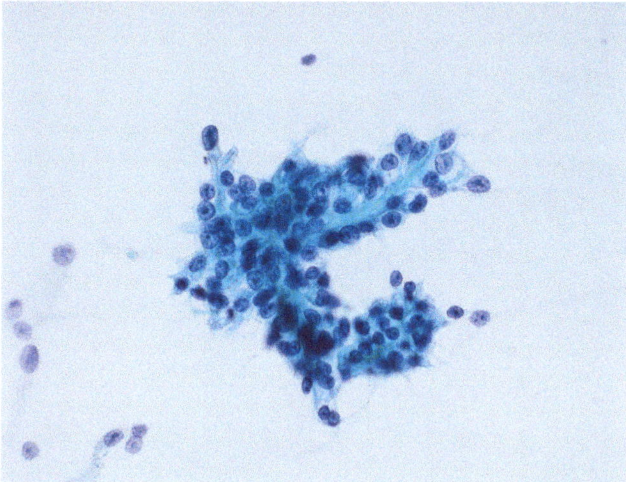

Fig. 2.11 Intraoperative smear (alcohol-fixed and Papanicolaou-stained) from cut surface of CCC, showing a papillary cluster of cells with large and variably sized nuclei with irregular chromatin clumping. Stromal hyalinization is present at the upper left, and several tumor cells contain clear cytoplasm

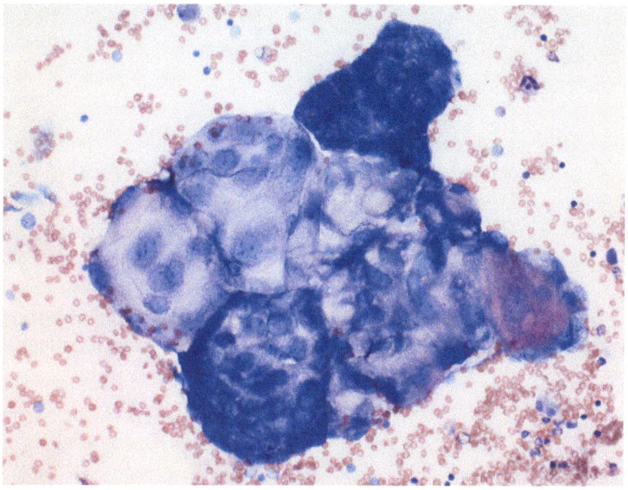

Fig. 2.13 Intraoperative smear (air-dried and Giemsa-stained) showing clusters of malignant cells with clear cytoplasm

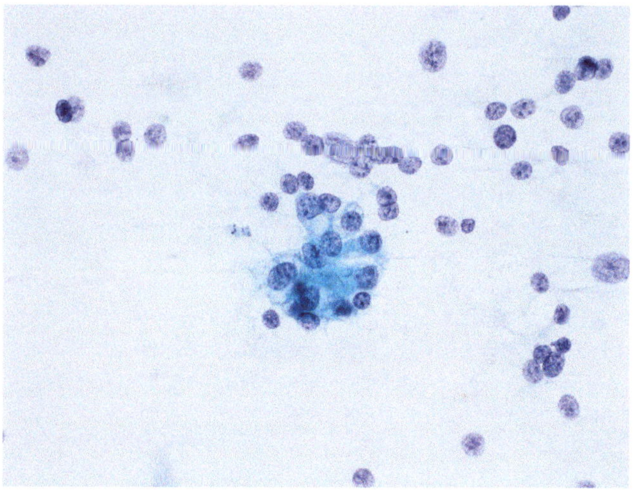

Fig. 2.12 Another intraoperative Papanicolaou-stained smear with micropapillary cluster of clear cells

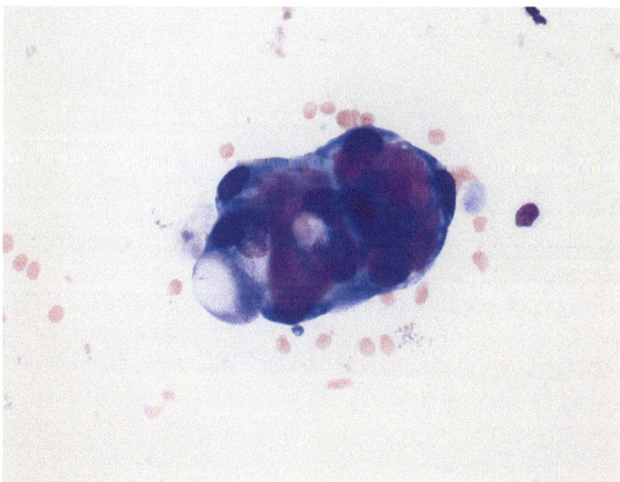

Fig. 2.14 Another intraoperative air-dried and Giemsa-stained smear with cluster of malignant clear cells

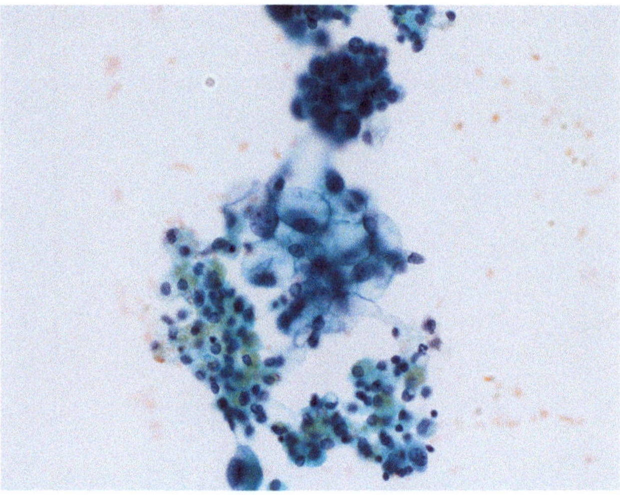

Fig. 2.15 Ascitic fluid smear showing central nest of large malignant clear cells in close proximity to two nests of small cohesive mesothelial cells

References

1. Heatley MK (2012) A systematic review of papers examining the use of intraoperative frozen section in predicting the final diagnosis of ovarian lesions. Int J Gynecol Pathol 31:111–115
2. Stewart CL, Brennan BA, Hammond IG et al (2008) Intraoperative assessment of clear cell carcinoma of the ovary. Int J Gynecol Pathol 27:475–482

Typical Histopathology

3

Clear cell carcinoma of the ovary is one of the most instantly recognizable ovarian tumors and probably the single most recognizable type of ovarian adenocarcinoma. In our own review of over six hundred cases, over 95 % of cases submitted as clear cell carcinoma (CCC) were accepted on histopathologic central review, and a similar proportion of the cases were accepted in a review done in Canada [1]. The picture at scanning lens magnification is one of micropapillary, tubulocystic, and solid patterns, often with admixtures of more than one of these patterns (and occasionally others as well) in the same tumor (Figs. 3.1, 3.2, 3.3, 3.4, 3.5, 3.6, 3.7, 3.8, 3.9, 3.10, 3.11, 3.12, 3.13, 3.14, 3.15, 3.16, 3.17, 3.18, and 3.19).

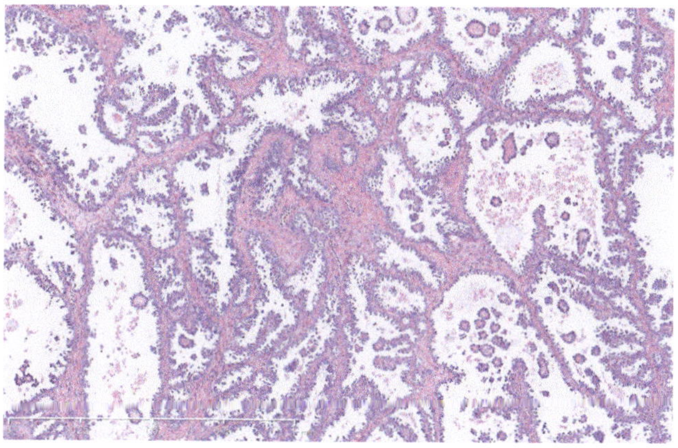

Fig. 3.1 Low-power magnification view of ovarian clear cell carcinoma (CCC) with predominantly micropapillary pattern. Micropapillae with largely hyalinized stroma grown into large cystic spaces

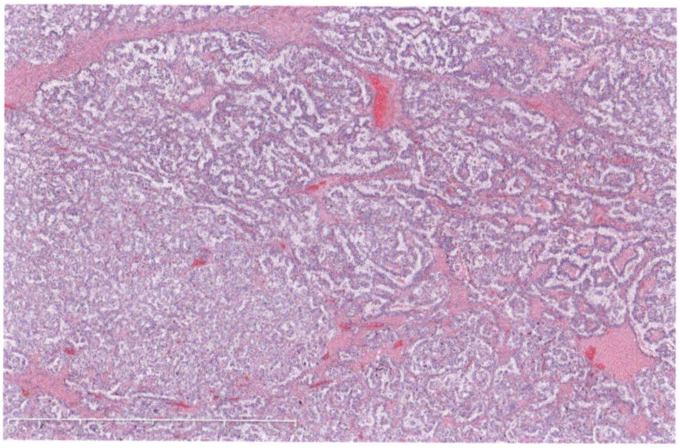

Fig. 3.2 Tubulo-papillary pattern in CCC, with admixture of micropapillary and tubular growth

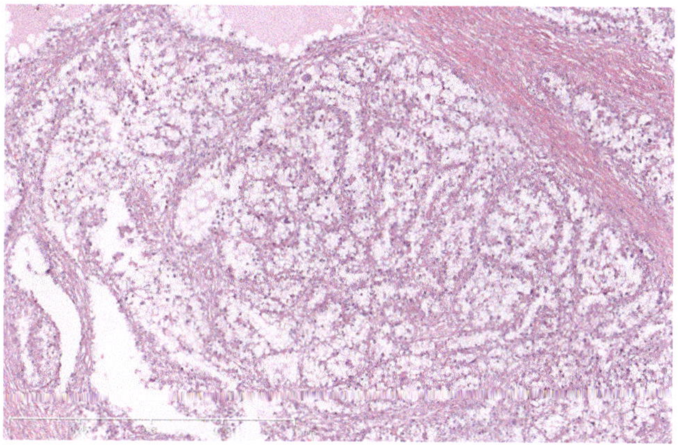

Fig. 3.3 Tubular pattern, with uniformly sized tubules lined by predominantly clear cells

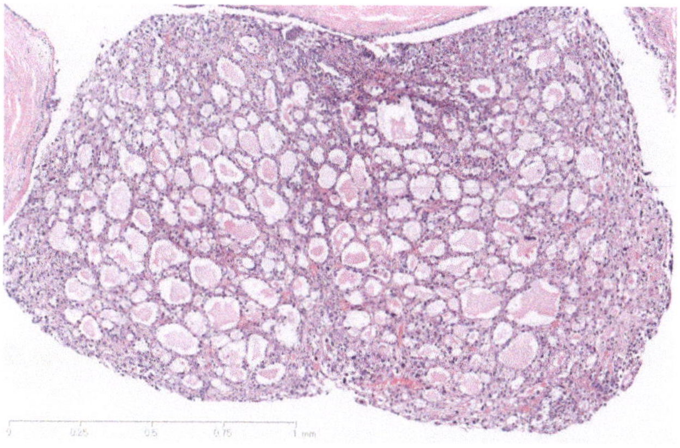

Fig. 3.4 Tubular pattern, with small tubules containing myxoid-appearing debris

J. Kigawa et al., *Atlas of Clear Cell Carcinoma of the Ovary: A Pathological Guide*,
DOI 10.1007/978-4-431-55438-7_3, © Springer Japan 2015

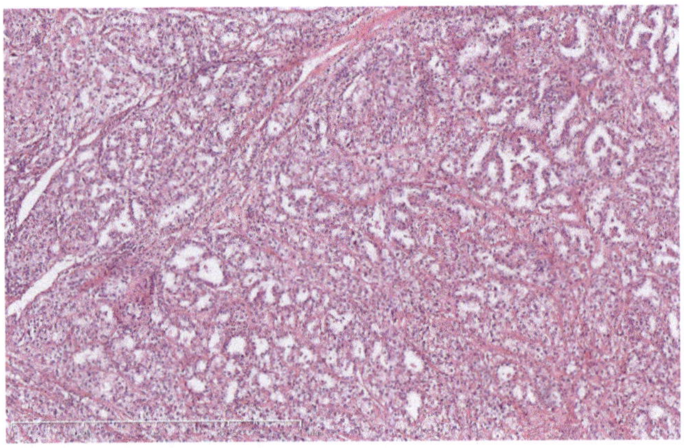

Fig. 3.5 Tubular pattern, in which there is more variation in tubular size and shape

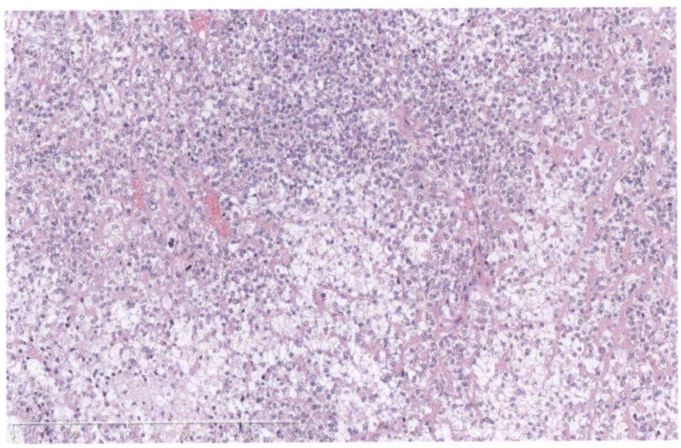

Fig. 3.6 Solid pattern of growth, in which clear cytoplasm can be seen in a good many but not all of the cells at this magnification

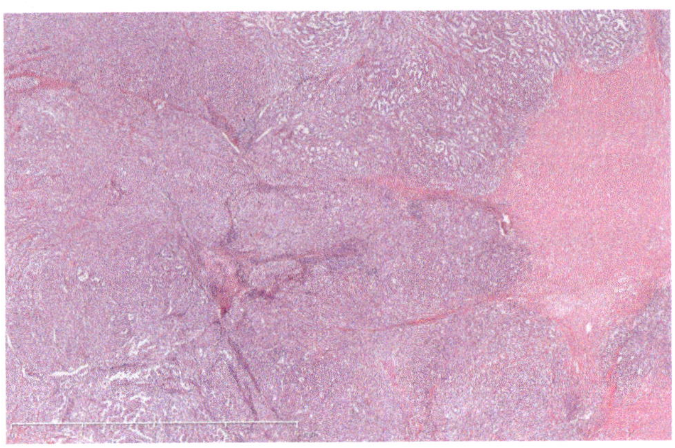

Fig. 3.7 Admixture of solid and tubular growth patterns

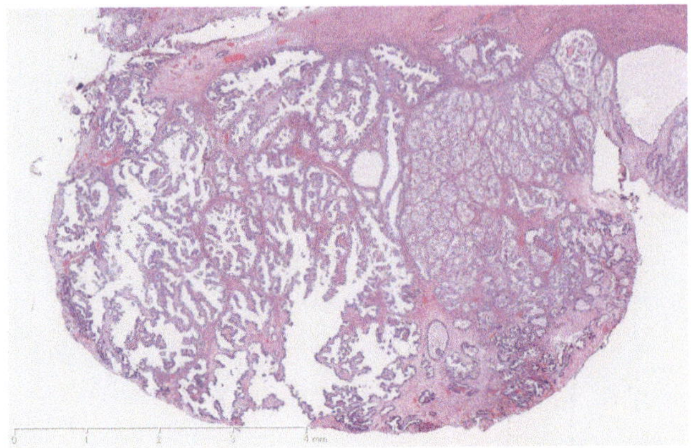

Fig. 3.8 Admixture of micropapillary and solid patterns

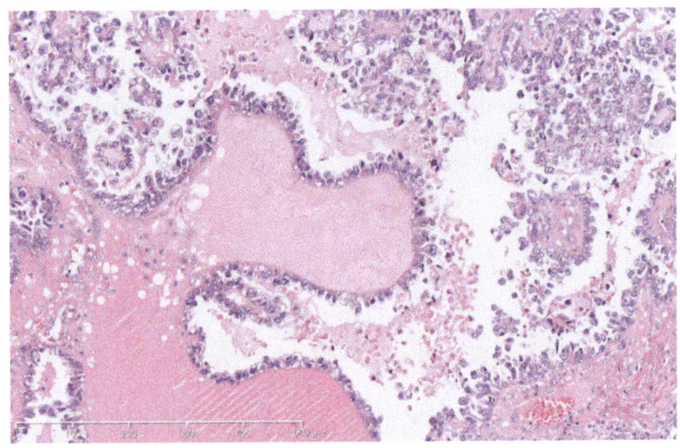

Fig. 3.9 Papillary growth of CCC featuring both macro- and micropapillae

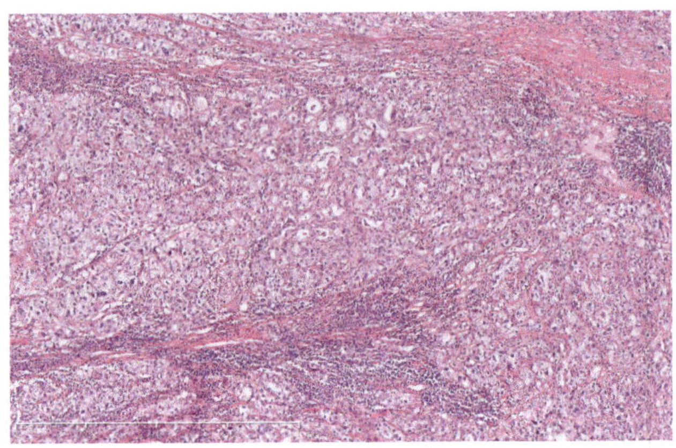

Fig. 3.10 Admixture of solid and tubular patterns in a predominantly fibrous stroma

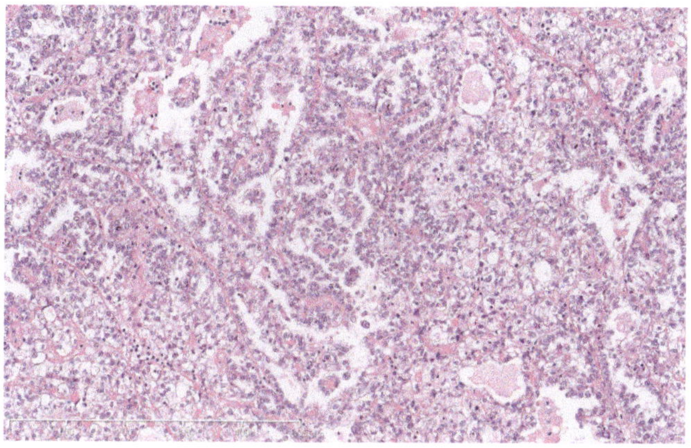

Fig. 3.11 Admixture in one field of tubular, micropapillary, and solid grown patterns

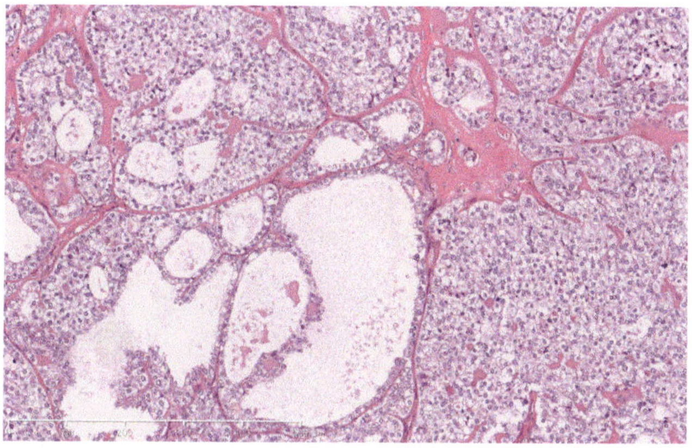

Fig. 3.12 Solid and tubulocystic growth patterns

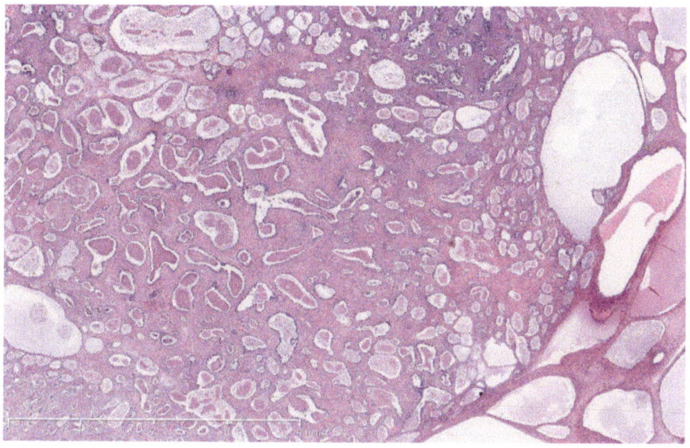

Fig. 3.13 Adenofibromatous pattern of CCC, in which both small and large tubules grow within a largely fibromatous stroma

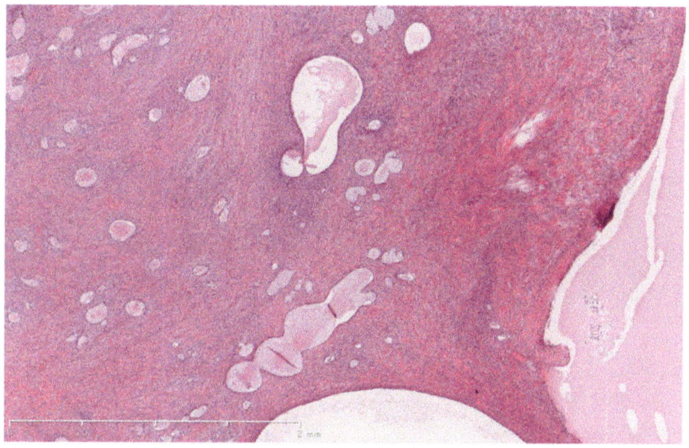

Fig. 3.14 Adenofibromatous pattern with more widely spaced tubules, some of which are cystically dilated, than in Fig. 3.13

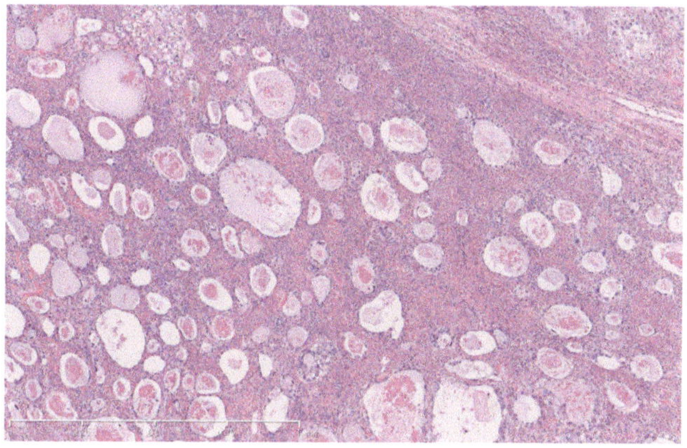

Fig. 3.15 Adenofibromatous pattern in which the tubules are separated by a more cellular fibrous stroma. Note the necrotic-appearing debris within tubular lumina

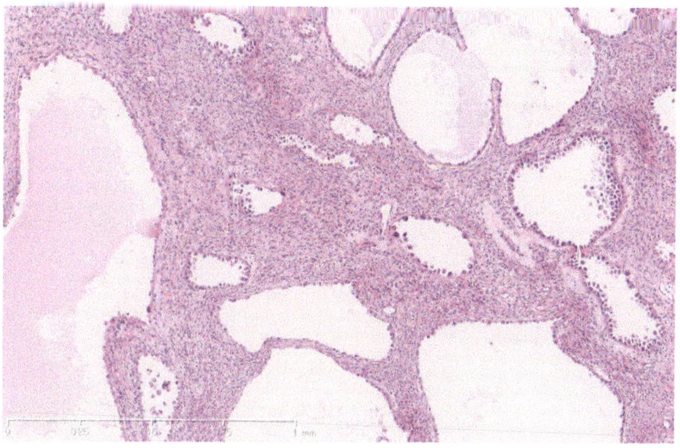

Fig. 3.16 Adenofibromatous pattern in which a cellular ovarian cortical-type stroma is present. Hobnail type cells are easily seen lining the tubules at this magnification

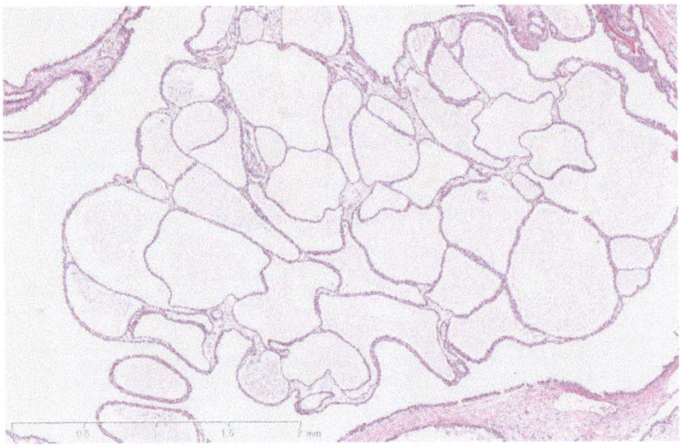

Fig. 3.17 Tubulocystic pattern in which the tubular structures are all cystic and minimal stroma remains between them

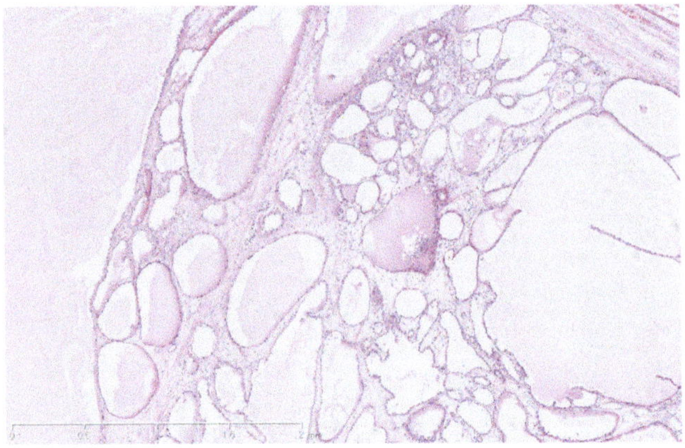

Fig. 3.18 Another tubulocystic growth pattern in which small tubules and larger cystically dilated ones coexist

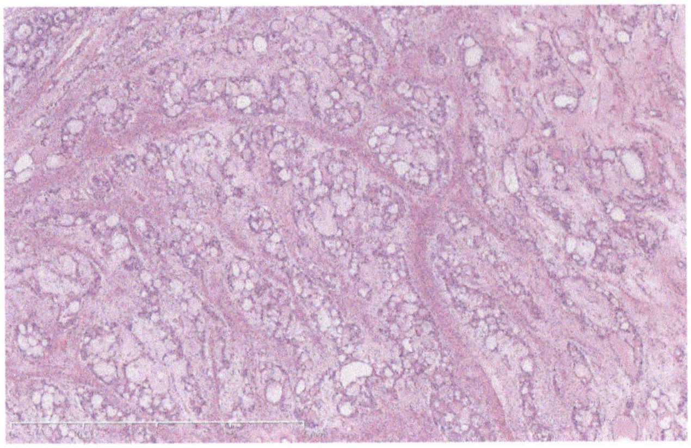

Fig. 3.19 Variant of tubulocystic pattern in which tubules have coalesced to create a cribriform growth pattern

The adenofibromatous pattern (Figs. 3.13, 3.14, 3.15, and 3.16) is present (alone or mixed with other patterns) in 20–25 % of cases. Atypia and evidence of stromal invasion are often minimal in these foci, leading to the differential diagnosis with benign or borderline clear cell adenofibroma. Multiple sections may be required for the diagnosis of CCC.

Stromal hyalinization is a prominent feature of almost all ovarian CCCs. This can vary from early and focal hyalinization within the stroma of micropapillae (Figs. 3.20 and 3.21) to more extensive stromal hyalinization in all patterns (Figs. 3.22, 3.23, 3.24, 3.25, 3.26, 3.27, 3.28, and 3.29), to fields or cases in which hyalinization has become so prominent that it is difficult to find typical tumor cells (Figs. 3.30 and 3.31).

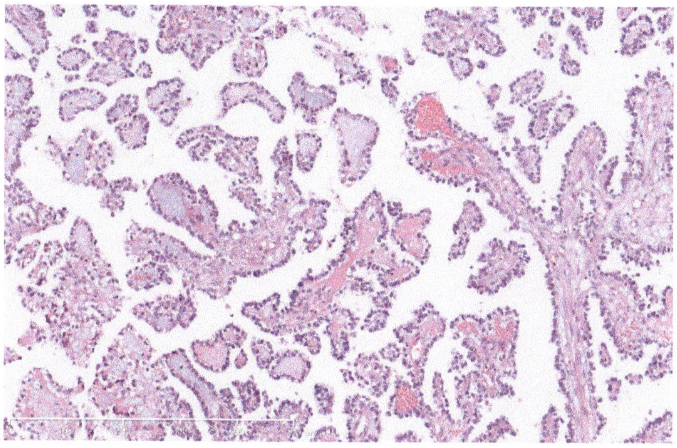

Fig. 3.20 Micropapillary CCC showing early hyalinization, some of which appears myxoid, within the papillary structures

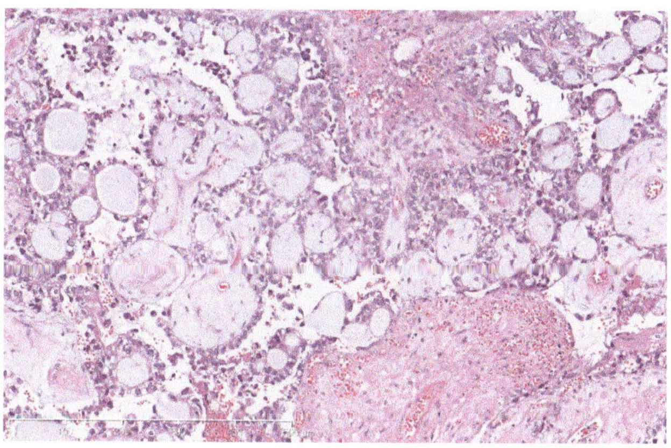

Fig. 3.21 More extensive hyalinization of micropapillae. Note the residual small compressed, or even vanished in this plane of section, vascular channels within the papillae

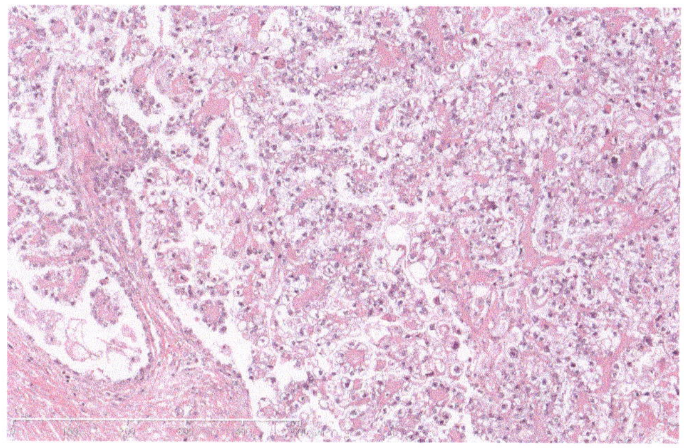

Fig. 3.22 Hyalinization predominantly of supporting stroma of a micropapillary and tubular CCC

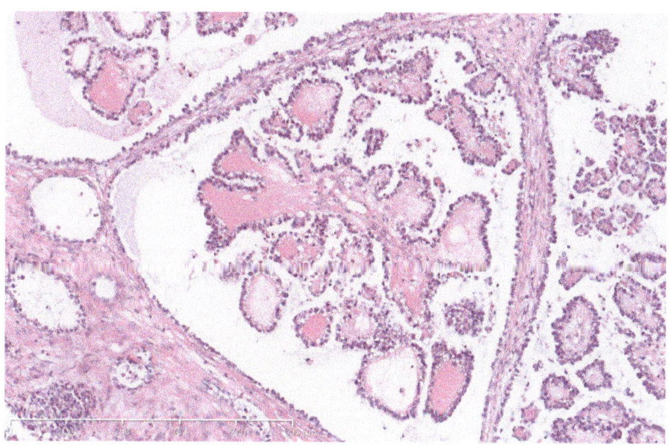

Fig. 3.23 More extensive hyalinization within micropapillae

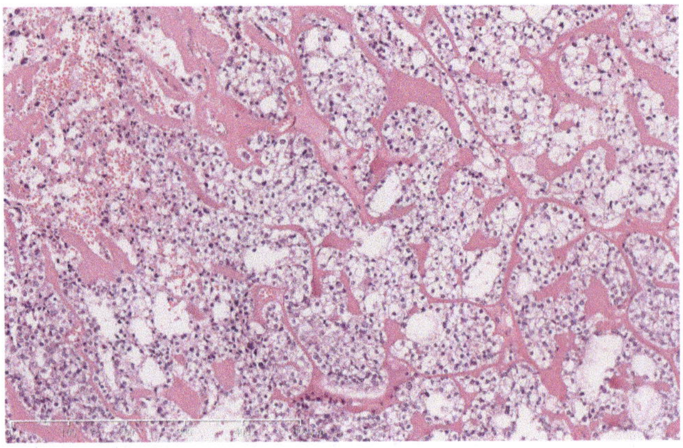

Fig. 3.24 Stromal hyalinization within a tubular and solid growth pattern

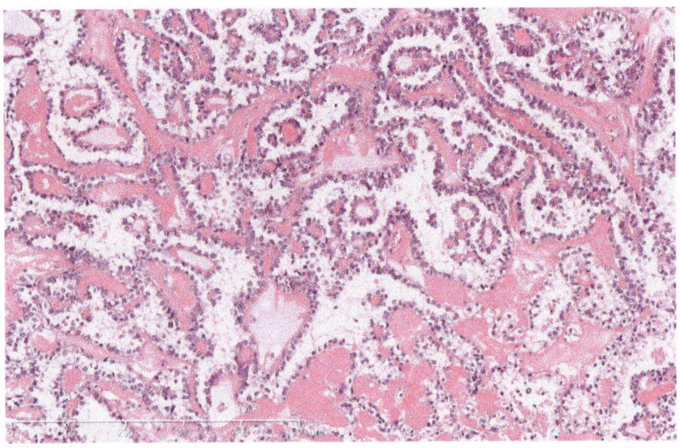

Fig. 3.25 Dense stromal hyalinization of a predominantly micropapillary focus of CCC

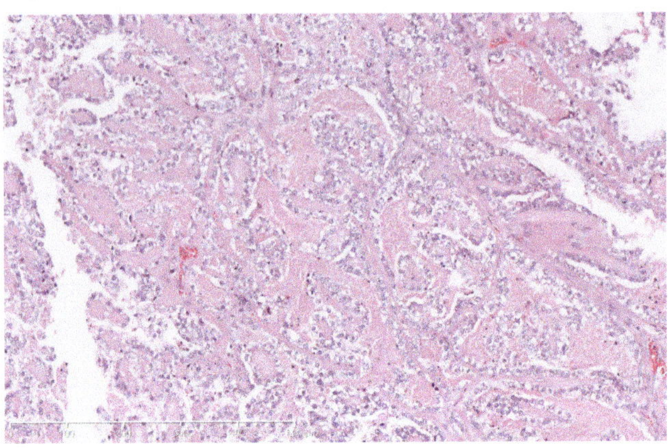

Fig. 3.26 More extensive stromal hyalinization in which, however, tumor cells are still clearly identifiable as clear cell type

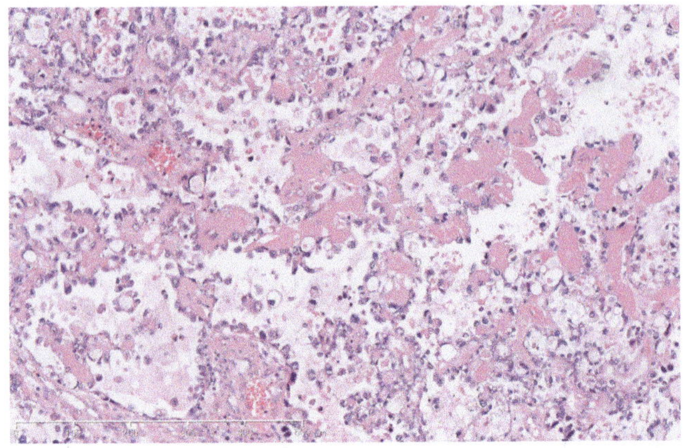

Fig. 3.27 Thick stromal hyalinization with residual predominantly hobnail cells

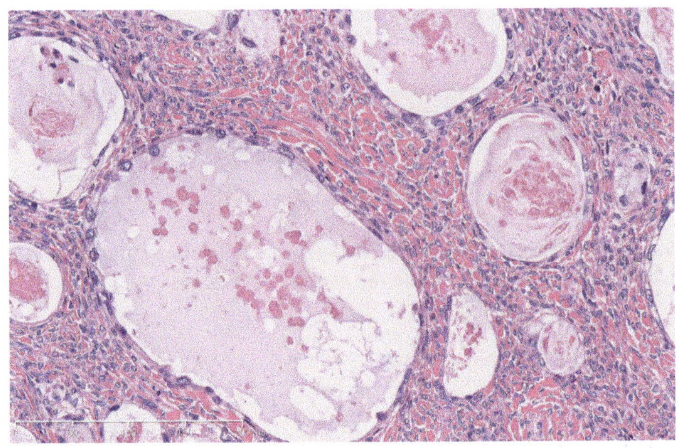

Fig. 3.28 Dense stromal hyalinization within an adenofibromatous type of CCC

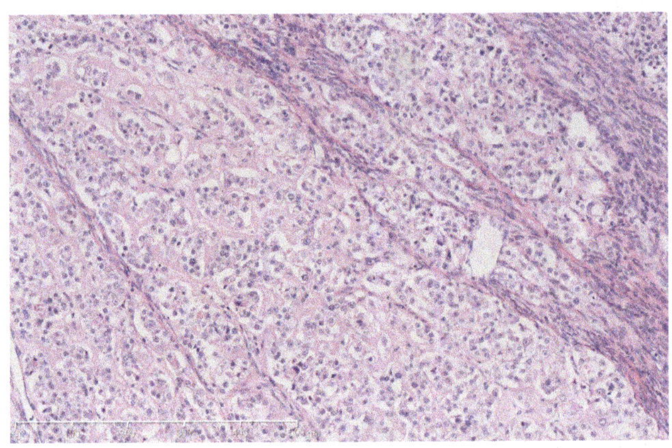

Fig. 3.29 Dense hyalinization in which tumor cells are compressed but still easily identifiable

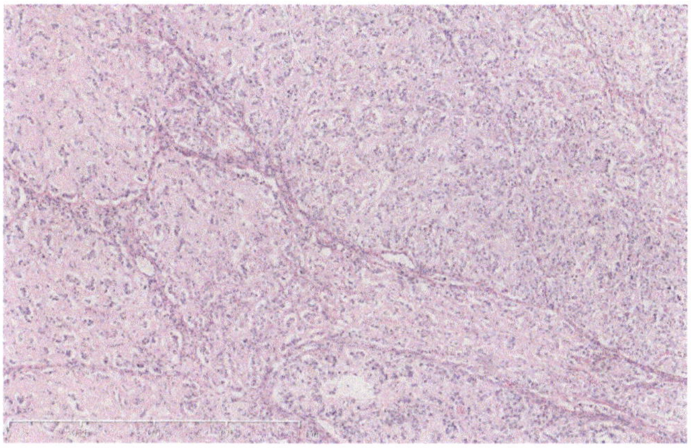

Fig. 3.30 In this hyalinized focus, the tumor cells are densely compressed and not identifiable as of any particular type

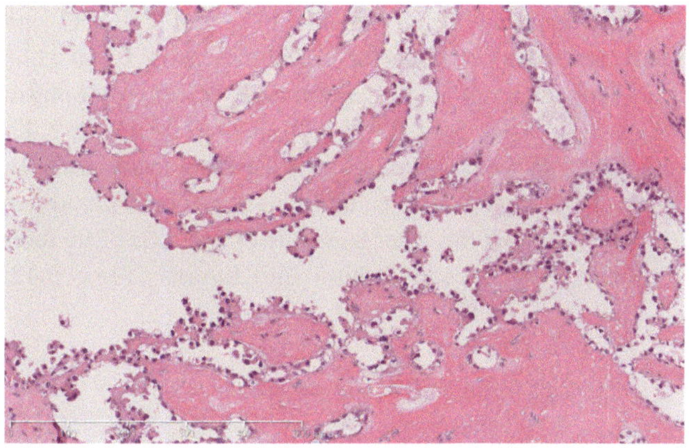

Fig. 3.31 Extensive stromal hyalinization with relatively few residual hobnail tumor cells

The dominant tumor cells of ovarian CCC are characterized as either clear or hobnail cells. Clear cells are characterized by voluminous clear cytoplasm (Figs. 3.32, 3.33, 3.34, 3.35, 3.36, 3.37, 3.38, 3.39, 3.40, and 3.41), in which the clarity of the cytoplasm has been shown to be the result of voluminous deposits of glycogen. Hobnail cells, on the other hand, are characterized by their projections in hobnail fashion into lumina (Figs. 3.42, 3.43, 3.44, 3.45, 3.46, 3.48, 3.49, and 3.50). Variable proportions of clear and hobnail cells are found in different CCCs, and the dominance of one or the other type has never been shown to be of prognostic significance. The hobnail cells may also contain large amounts of clear cytoplasm (Figs. 3.42 and 3.43), but more often the nuclear/cytoplasmic ratios of these cells are high because of relatively small amounts of cytoplasm.

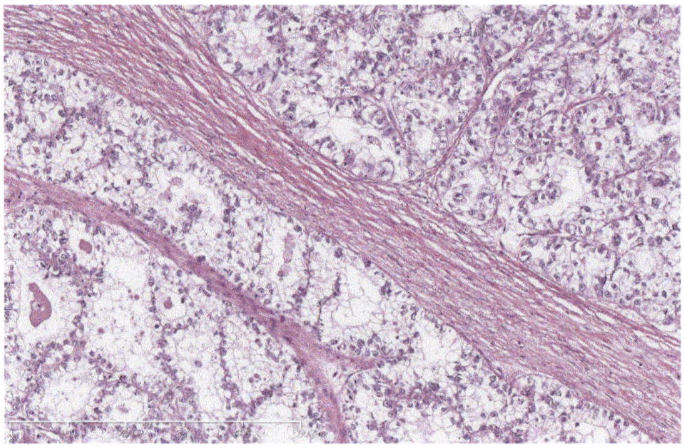

Fig. 3.32 Clear cell carcinoma field composed exclusively of clear cells, containing voluminous optically clear cytoplasm

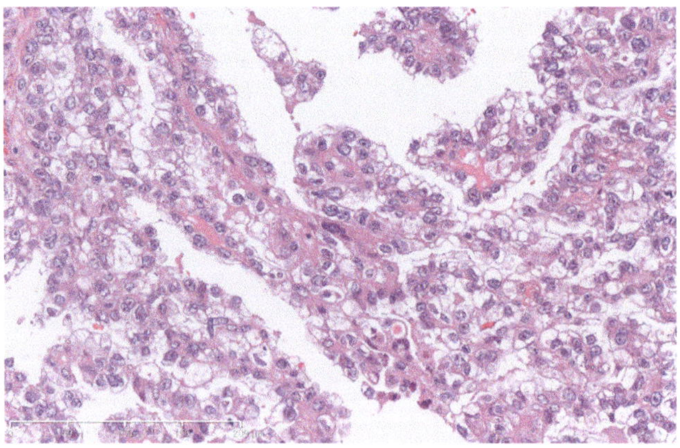

Fig. 3.33 Another field composed exclusively of clear cells with a somewhat higher nuclear/cytoplasmic ratio

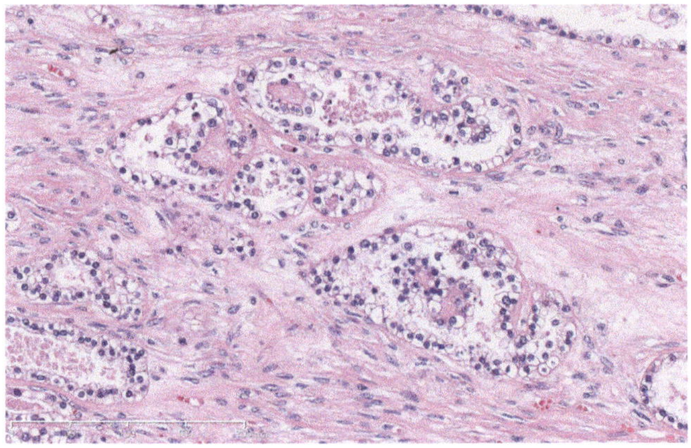

Fig. 3.34 Clear cells in a tubulocystic growth pattern

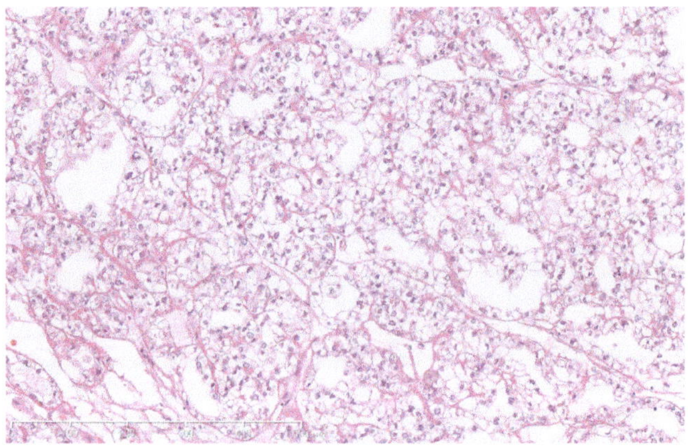

Fig. 3.35 Clear cells in a tubulocystic and solid growth pattern

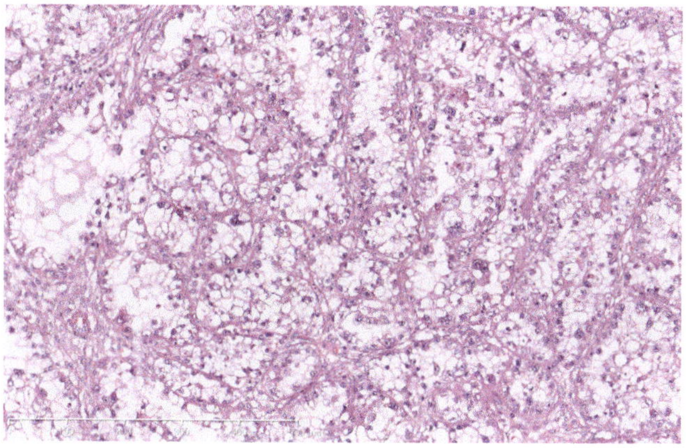

Fig. 3.36 Clear cells in a tubulocystic pattern

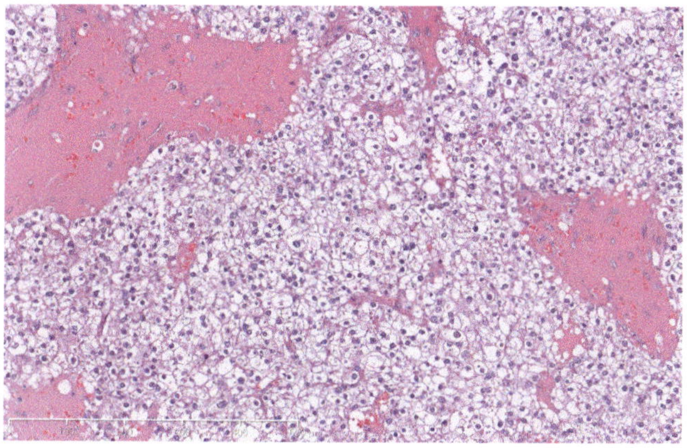

Fig. 3.37 Solid focus composed exclusively of clear cells

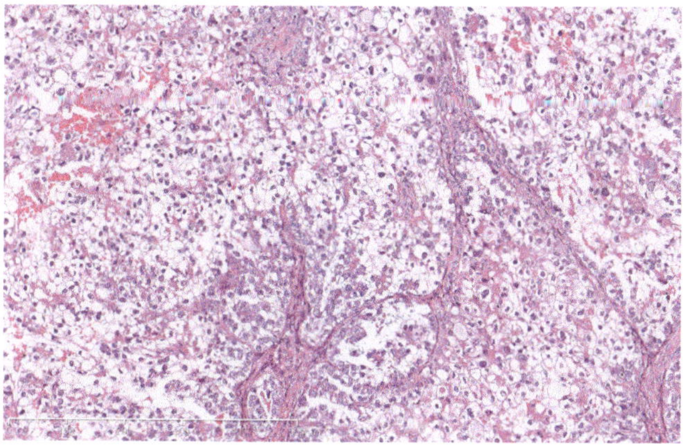

Fig. 3.38 Predominantly solid focus of clear cells. Note significant nuclear atypia even at this low magnification

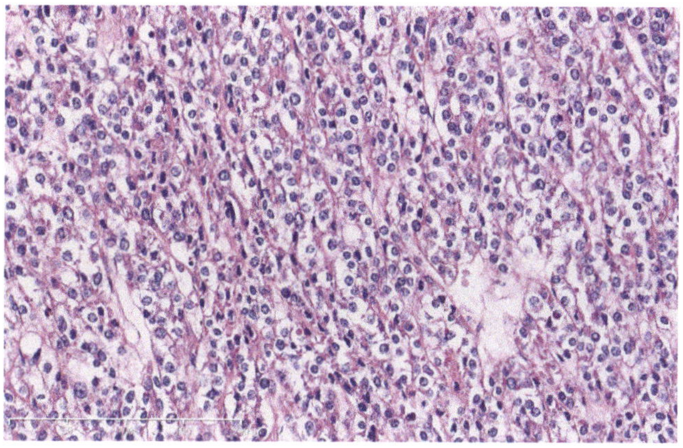

Fig. 3.39 Clear cells in compressed tubules which lack residual lumina, thus being classified as a solid growth pattern

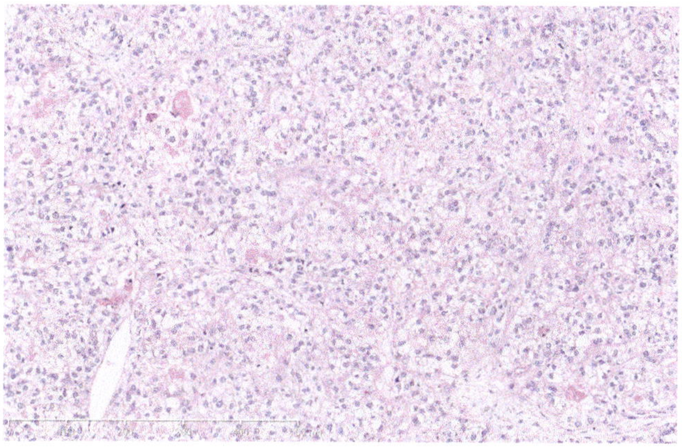

Fig. 3.40 Clear cells in a solid growth pattern

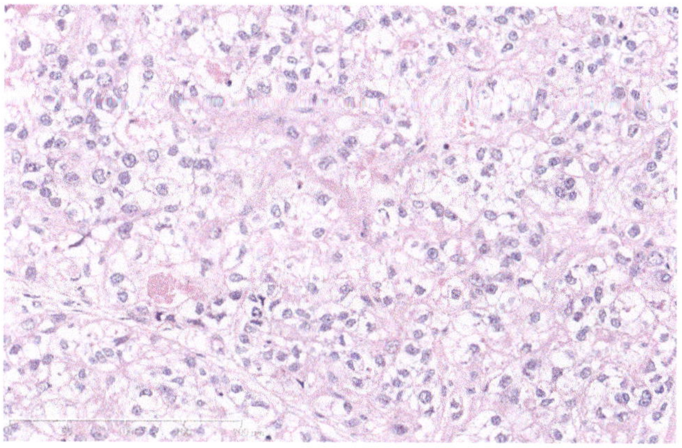

Fig. 3.41 Higher-power view of clear cells in a solid growth pattern. Note nuclear atypia in this field

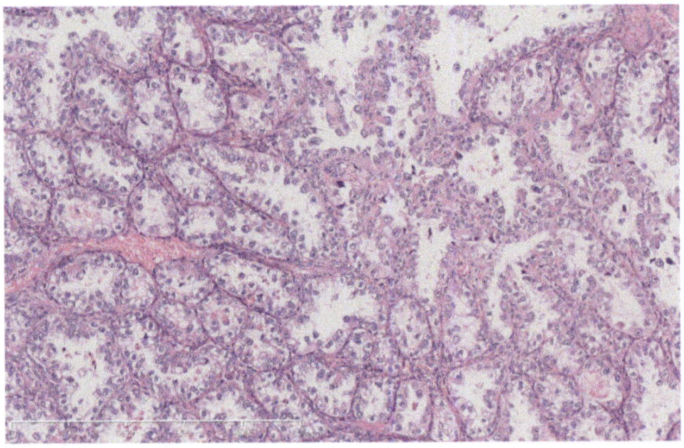

Fig. 3.42 Tubulocystic pattern of growth with hobnail cells projecting into lumina. Most of the hobnail cells in this field also contain clear cytoplasm

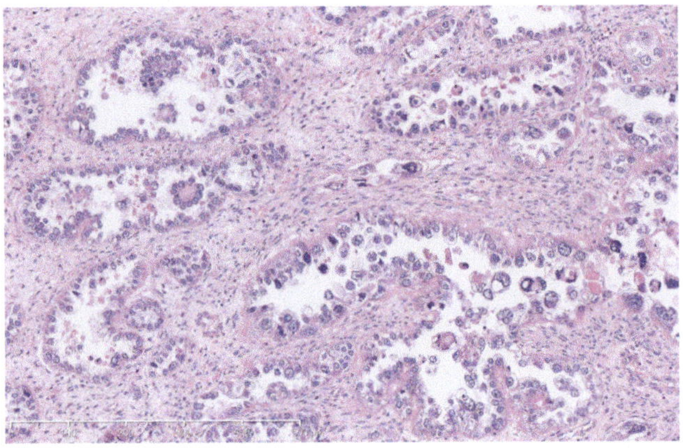

Fig. 3.43 Hobnail cells, many of which contain clear cytoplasm, at higher magnification

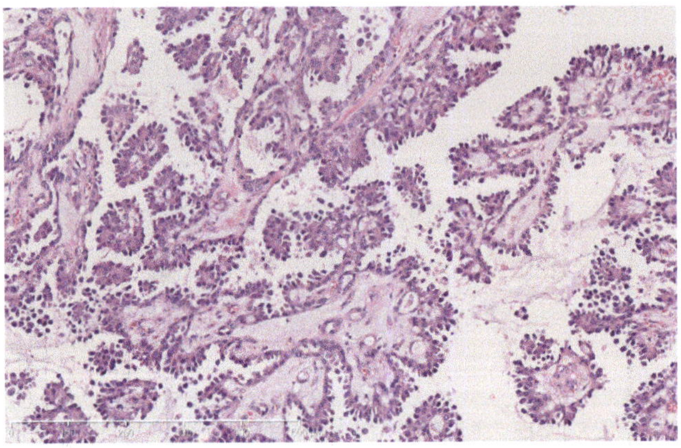

Fig. 3.44 Micropapillary CCC lined by hobnail cells without clear cytoplasm. The hobnail pattern is well visualized even at this relatively low magnification by the presence of individual cells projecting into the lumen

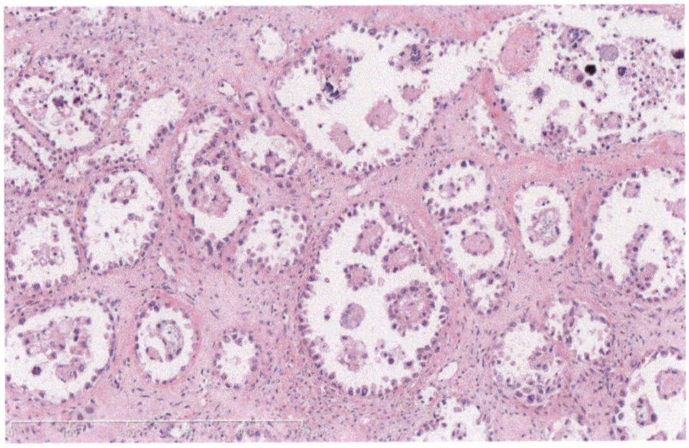

Fig. 3.45 Micropapillary CCC lined predominantly by hobnail cells

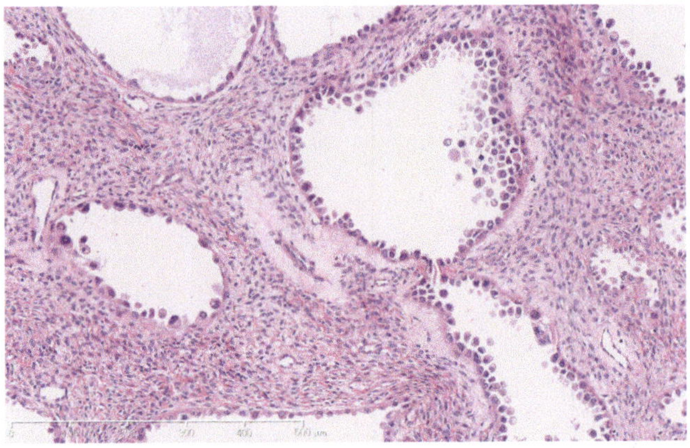

Fig. 3.46 Adenofibromatous type of CCC with hobnail cells lining the tubules

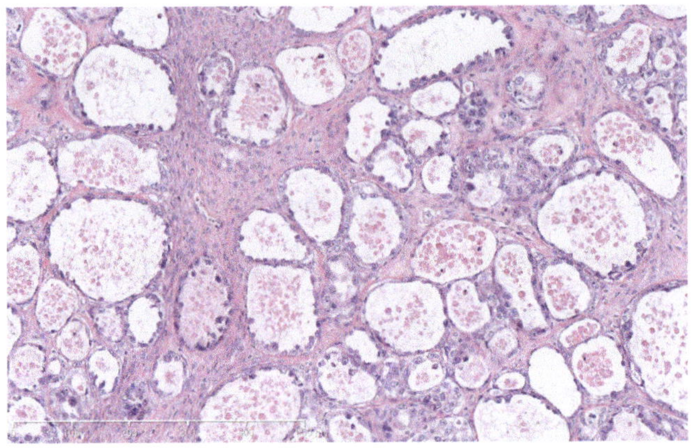

Fig. 3.47 Another adenofibromatous pattern with hobnail cells

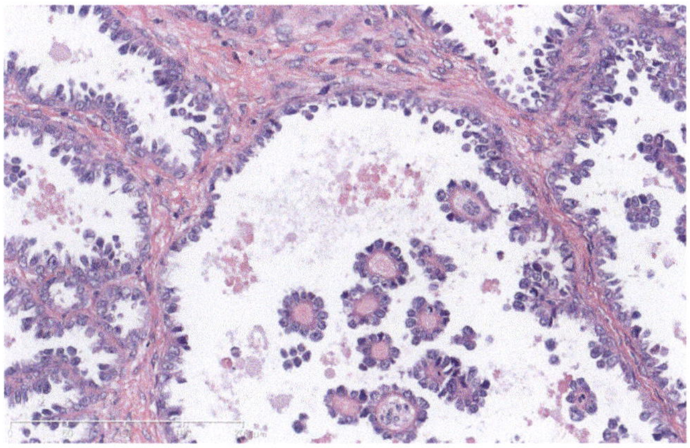

Fig. 3.48 Micropapillary and tubular pattern with individual hobnail cells projecting into lumina. The cytoplasmic content of the cells appears to be minimal

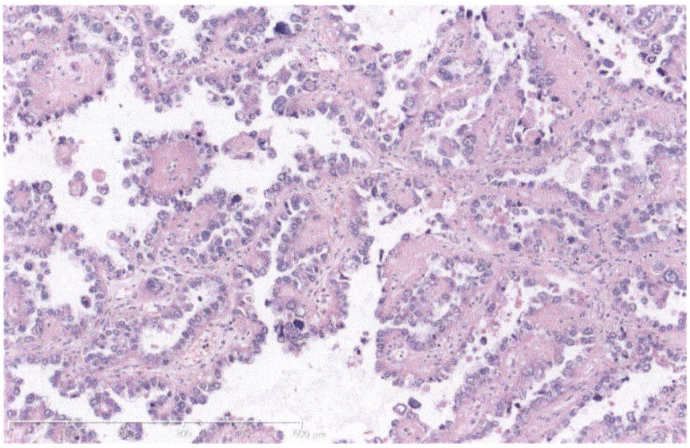

Fig. 3.49 More hobnail cells at higher magnification. A few of these also have clear cytoplasm

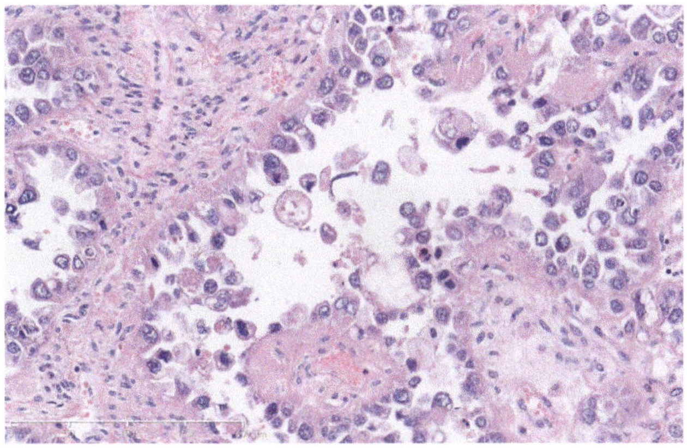

Fig. 3.50 High-power view of a hobnail cell field of CCC. One cell appears to be in mitosis, a rare finding in these tumors. Nuclear atypia is prominent

Bizarre nuclear atypia is a characteristic feature of ovarian CCC and may be focal or diffuse (Figs. 3.51, 3.52, 3.53, 3.54, 3.55, 3.56, 3.57, 3.58, and 3.59). The atypical nuclei generally have a malignant appearance, but in some cells, they may appear degenerative. Nuclear atypia is, of course, seen in many other ovarian cancers, but the distinctive feature of ovarian CCC is the combination of marked atypia and minimal mitotic activity. A mitotic count greater than 5 per 10 high-power fields is almost never encountered, and most tumors will have mitotic counts between 0 and 2 per 10 HPF. Indeed, if one is tempted to diagnose CCC in an ovarian tumor with easily identifiable mitotic figures, one should think again about this diagnosis.

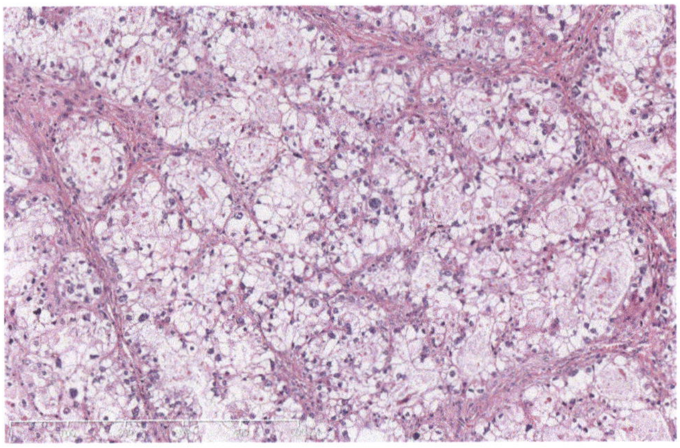

Fig. 3.51 Medium-power view of CCC in which numerous enlarged, hyperchromatic, atypical nuclei are easily identified

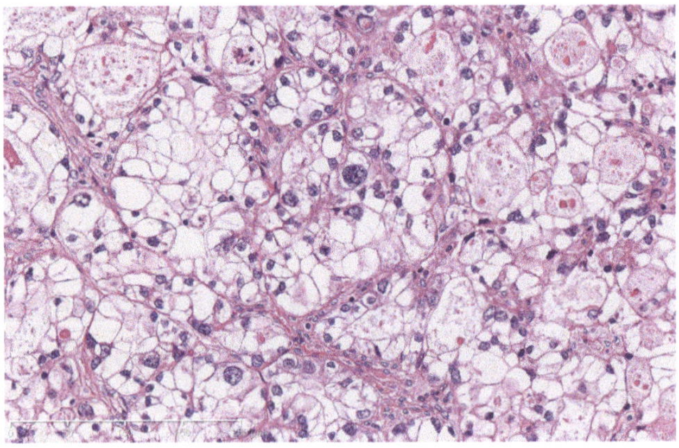

Fig. 3.52 Higher-power view of same field showing numerous large bizarre nuclei

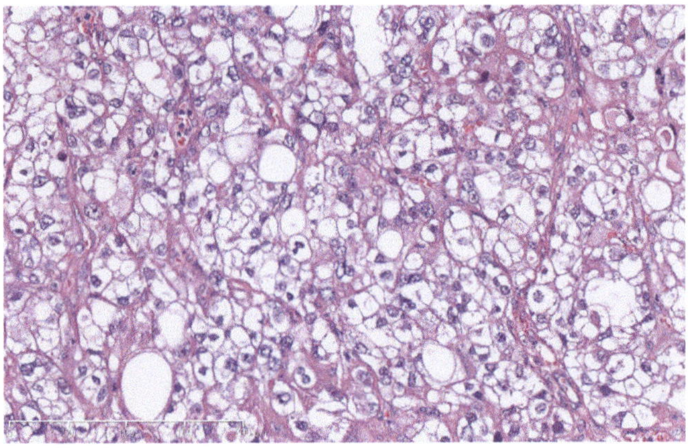

Fig. 3.53 Another case in which the cells have clear cytoplasm and numerous atypical nuclei

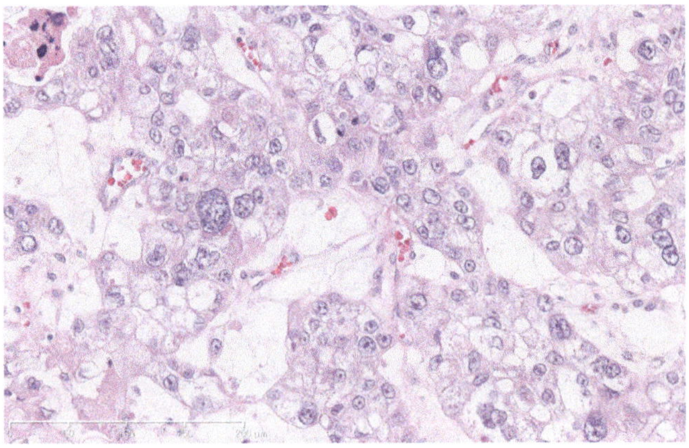

Fig. 3.54 In this case, the variation in nuclear size is almost tenfold, and irregular nuclear borders, clumped chromatin, and prominent nucleoli are easily identifiable

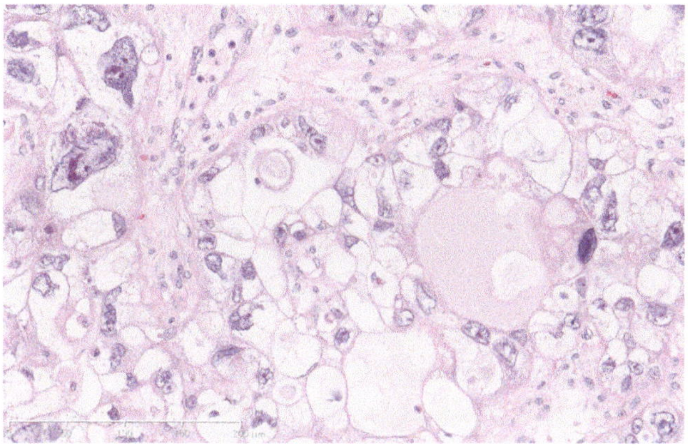

Fig. 3.55 Bizarre nuclei are seen in this clear cell field

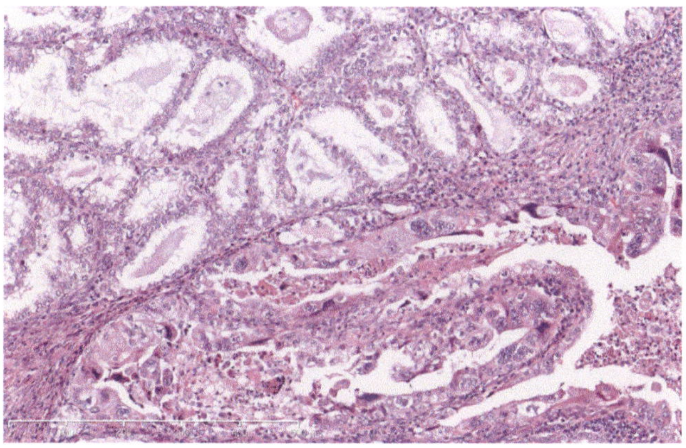

Fig. 3.56 In this field, the bizarre nuclear atypia is focal

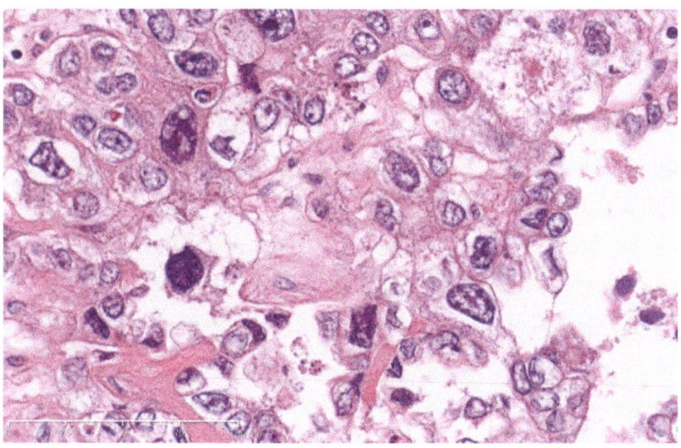

Fig. 3.57 Higher-power view showing numerous bizarre nuclei. Even the nuclei which are relatively uniform in size and shape are clearly atypical

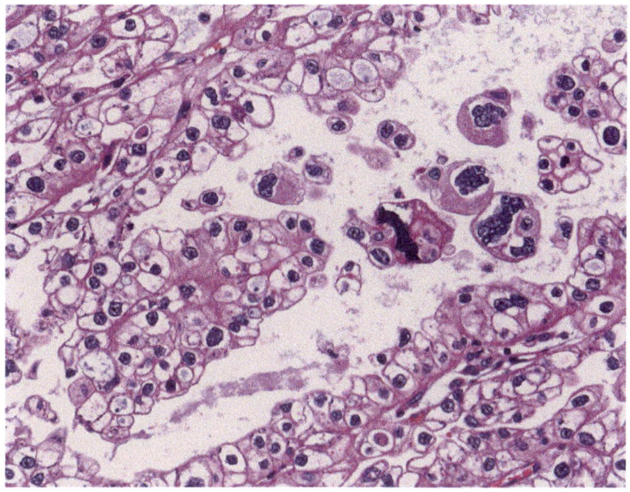

Fig. 3.58 Clear cell field with several bizarre nuclei which may be degenerative, but other nuclei in the field are also atypical

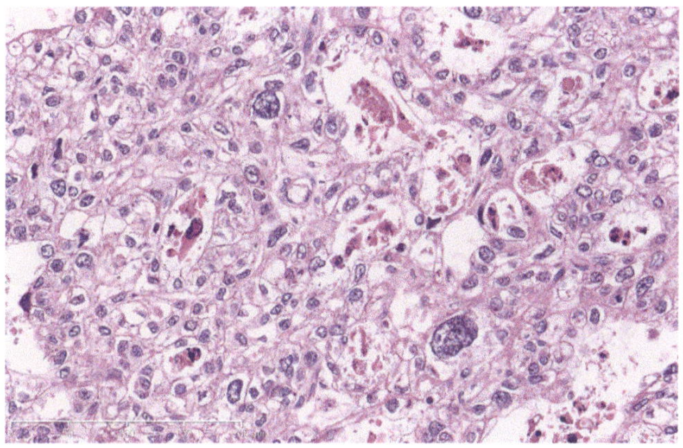

Fig. 3.59 Clear cell focus with great variation in nuclear size and shape and presence of two monstrous nuclei

Reference

1. Kobel M, Kalloger SE, Baker PM et al (2010) Diagnosis of ovarian carcinoma cell type is highly reproducible: a transcanadian study. Am J Surg Pathol 34:984–993

4 Histopathologic Variations

Oxyphilic differentiation is seen at least focally in at least half of ovarian CCCs, is prominent in 25–30 %, and may be the dominant (or occasionally the only) cell type in 5 % or less. The oxyphil cells, as in other tumors and other organs, are characterized by large quantities of amphophilic cytoplasm, often with enlarged atypical nuclei, and generally with no mitotic activity (Figs. 4.1, 4.2, 4.3, 4.4, 4.5, 4.6, 4.7, 4.8, 4.9, 4.10, 4.11, 4.12, and 4.13). These cells may be oncocytes, but they have never been shown to be packed with mitochondria like true oncocytes. In many instances, clear cells are seen adjacent to oxyphil cells, and some cells even have admixtures of clear and oxyphilic cytoplasm (Figs. 4.8, 4.9, 4.10, 4.11, 4.12, and 4.13).

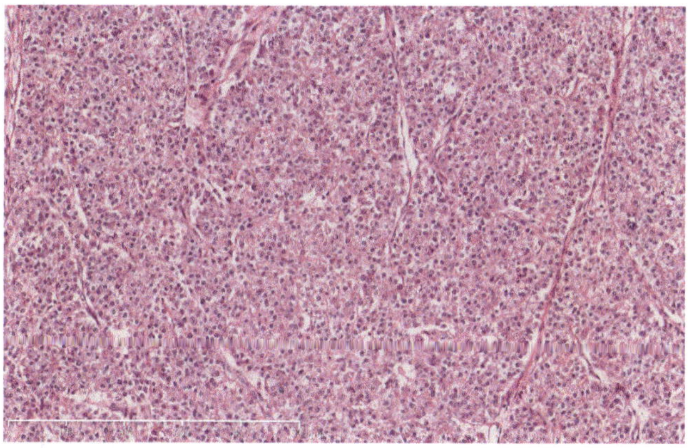

Fig. 4.1 Solid field within an ovarian CCC consisting exclusively of oxyphil cells

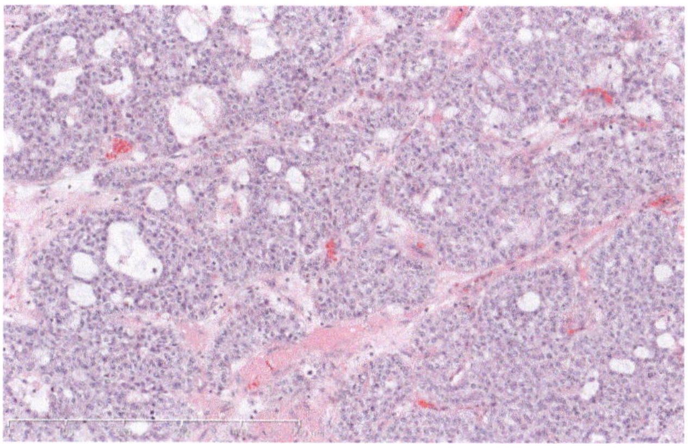

Fig. 4.2 Another tumor with another broad field of oxyphil cells

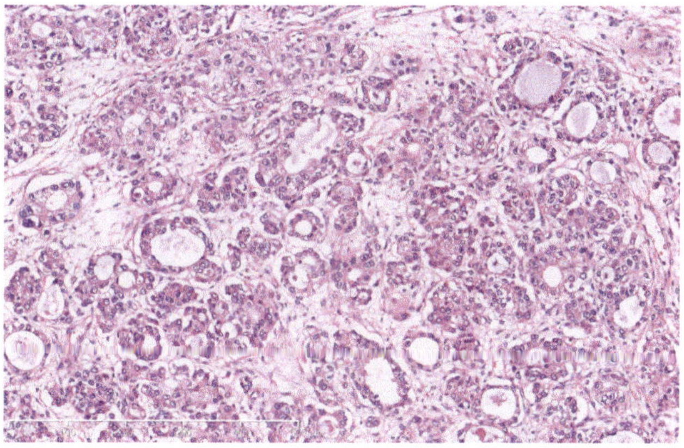

Fig. 4.3 At higher magnification, the amphophilic cytoplasm of these oxyphil cells is easily noted

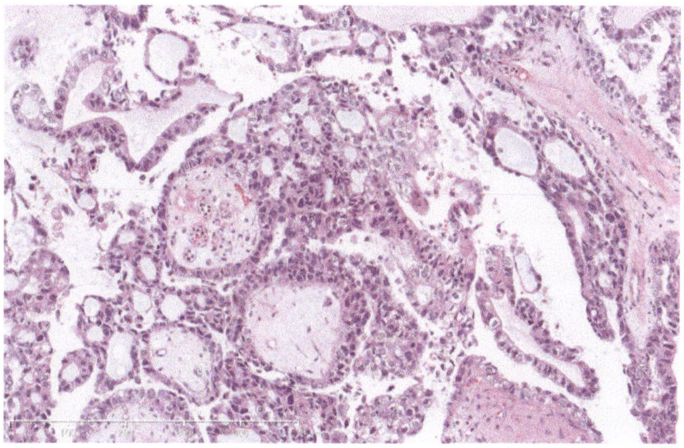

Fig. 4.4 Predominantly micropapillary and tubulocystic CCC with a field consisting exclusively of oxyphil differentiation

J. Kigawa et al., *Atlas of Clear Cell Carcinoma of the Ovary: A Pathological Guide*,
DOI 10.1007/978-4-431-55438-7_4, © Springer Japan 2015

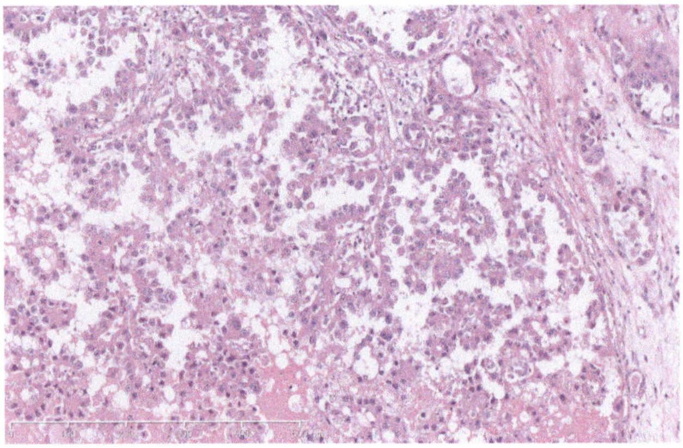

Fig. 4.5 Another pure oxyphil cells field in a CCC

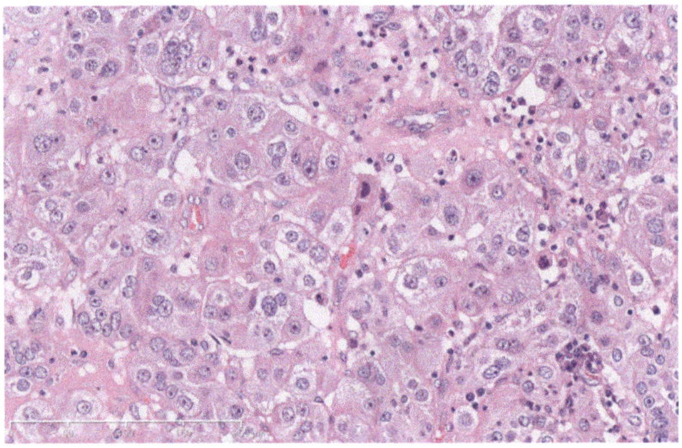

Fig. 4.6 Higher-power magnification of amphophilic, granular-appearing cytoplasm within oxyphil cells. Also note nuclear atypia

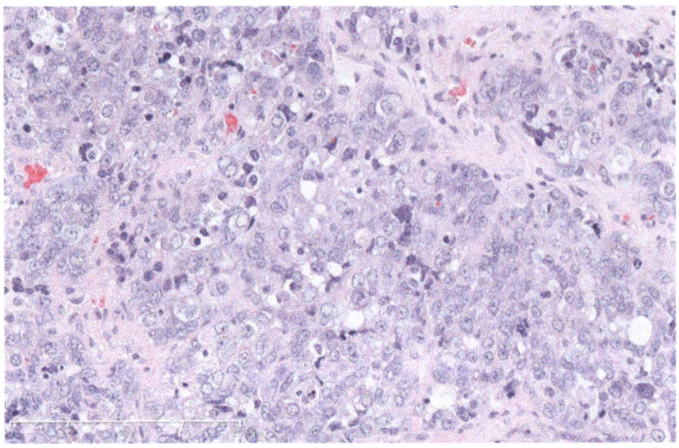

Fig. 4.7 Solid field of oxyphil cells infiltrated by some lymphocytes and plasma cells

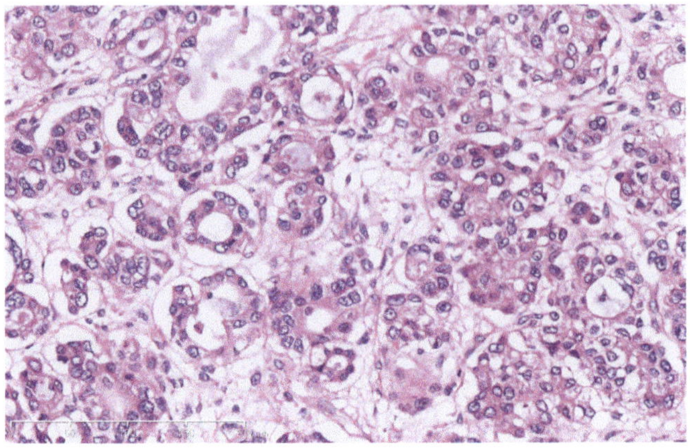

Fig. 4.8 Tumor field in which many individual cells show transitions from clear to oxyphilic cytoplasm

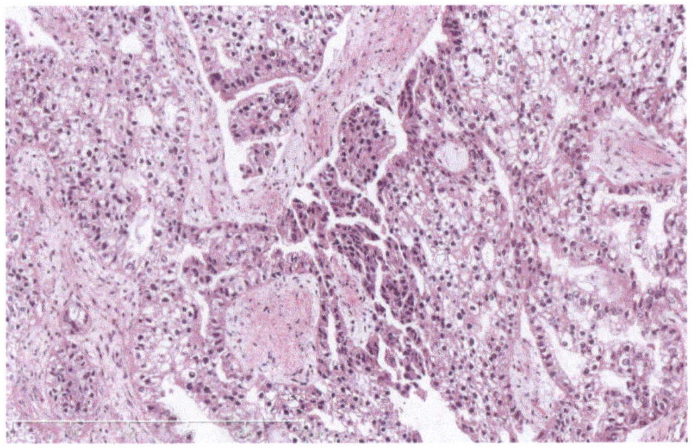

Fig. 4.9 Field in which oxyphil cells at the center are surrounded by clear cells on both sides, with some individual cells in transition

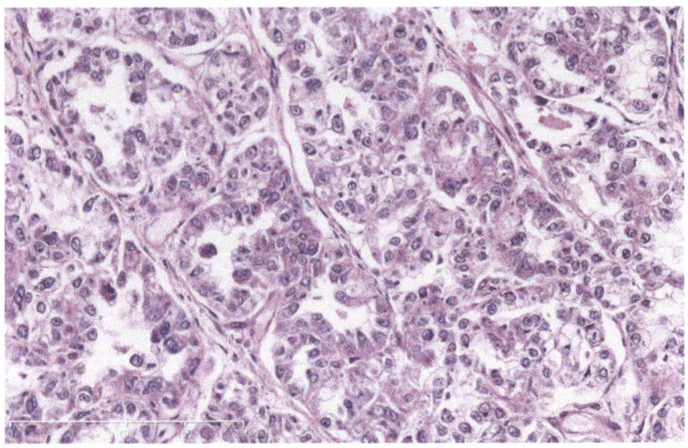

Fig. 4.10 Higher-power view of a tumor field in which individual cells show both oxyphilic and clear cell features

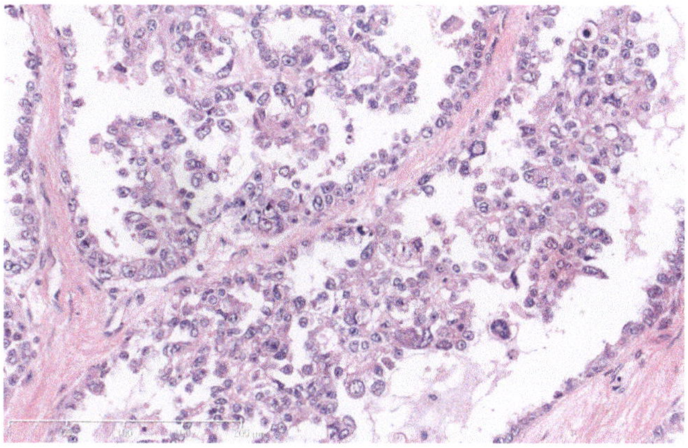

Fig. 4.11 Another tumor containing cells intermediate between clear cells and oxyphil cells

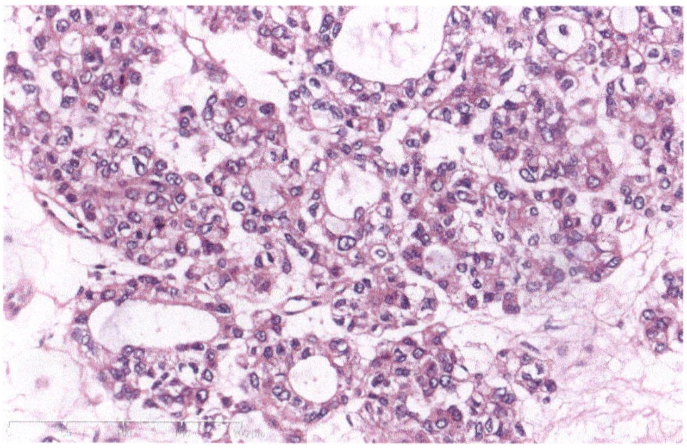

Fig. 4.12 More "hybrid" oxyphil/clear cells in a CCC

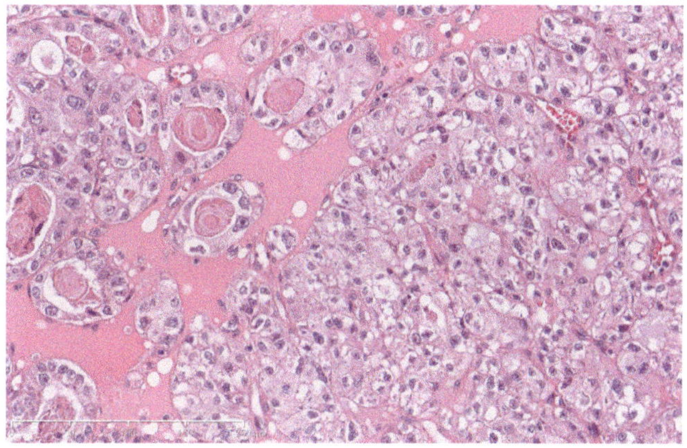

Fig. 4.13 Another tumor with cells showing both clear and oxyphilic features

Signet ring cells (Figs. 4.14, 4.15, 4.16, 4.17, and 4.18) are frequently present in small numbers but in our material were prominent in less than 10 % of cases. The intracytoplasmic inclusions may appear clear (Fig. 4.16), mucoid (Fig. 4.17), eosinophilic (Figs. 4.14 and 4.15), or basophilic (Fig. 4.18) in hematoxylin- and eosin (H&E)-stained preparations and usually compress the nucleus to one side of the cell.

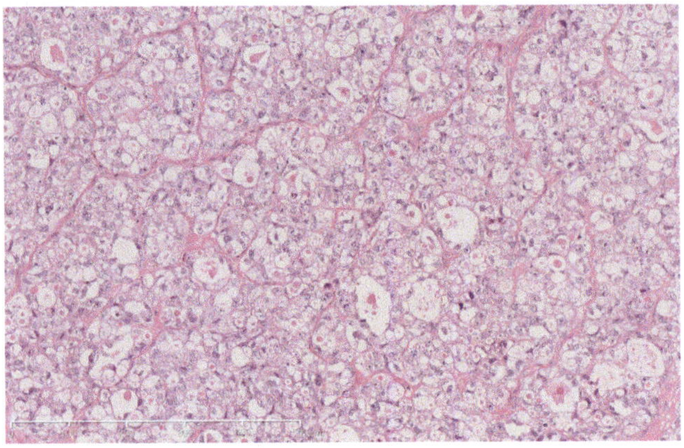

Fig. 4.14 Numerous signet ring cells (SRCs) containing eosinophilic globular inclusions

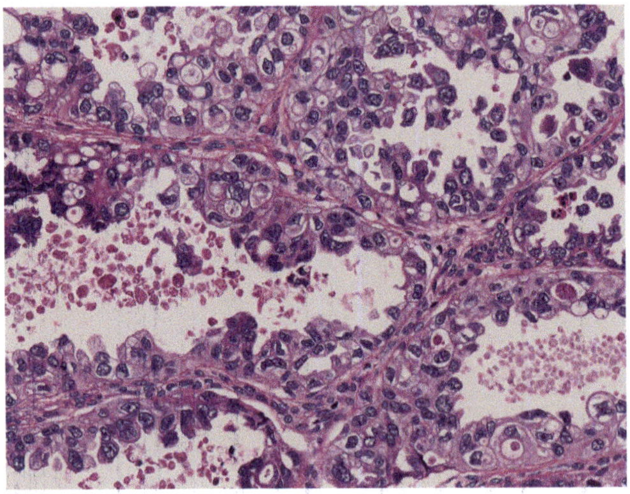

Fig. 4.15 Solid CCC field composed predominantly of SRCs with eosinophilic inclusions

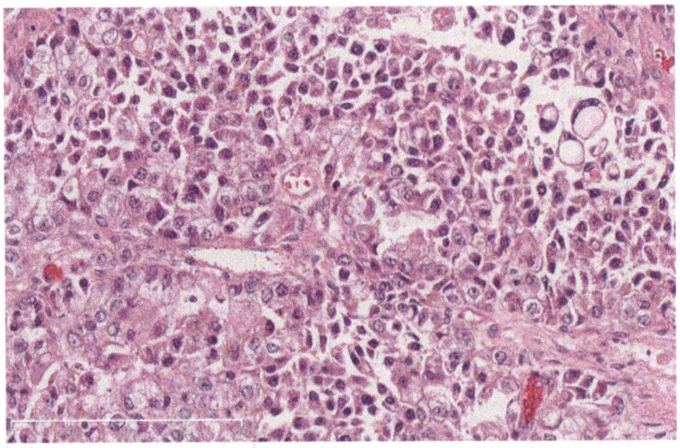

Fig. 4.16 The SRCs in this CCC appear to contain clear inclusions

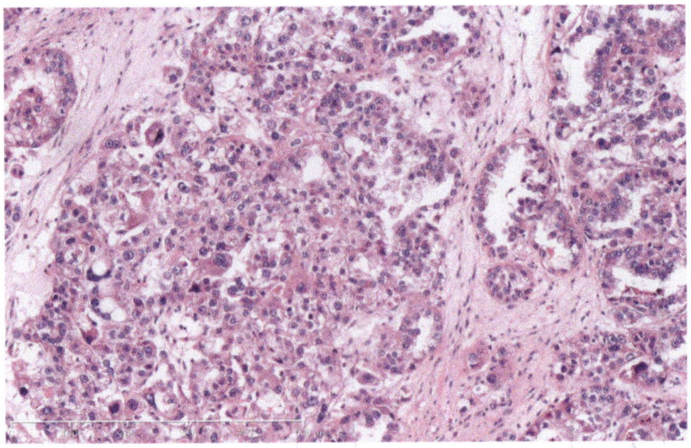

Fig. 4.17 Large mucoid-appearing inclusions compress the nuclei in these SRCs

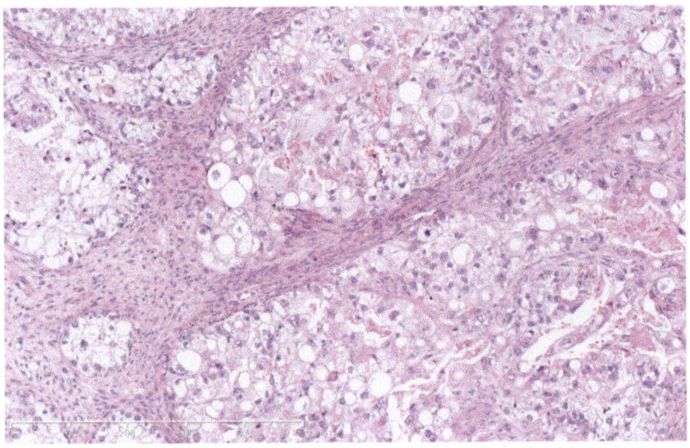

Fig. 4.18 These SRC inclusions are more basophilic

Another common finding in cases of ovarian CCC is endometriosis. In our series, 43 % of all cases could be shown to coexist with endometriosis in the same ovary, and in most cases, a direct origin could be demonstrated [1]. Among our cases which were associated with endometriosis, 69 % of the endometriotic regions were at least focally atypical and thus diagnosable as atypical endometriosis. Similar numbers have been reported in another review [2], in which endometriosis and its atypical variant were more common in cystic than in adenofibromatous CCCs. Examples of CCC arising in endometriosis and atypical endometriosis are shown in Figs. 4.19, 4.20, 4.21, 4.22, 4.23, 4.24, 4.25, 4.26, and 4.27.

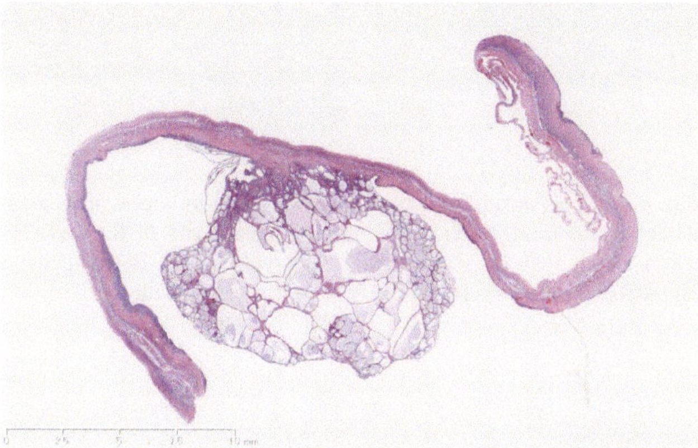

Fig. 4.19 Cases of CCC arising in endometriosis often present grossly and at lowest microscopic magnification as a ball of tumor within a cyst, as seen here. The cyst on closer examination turns out to be endometriosis

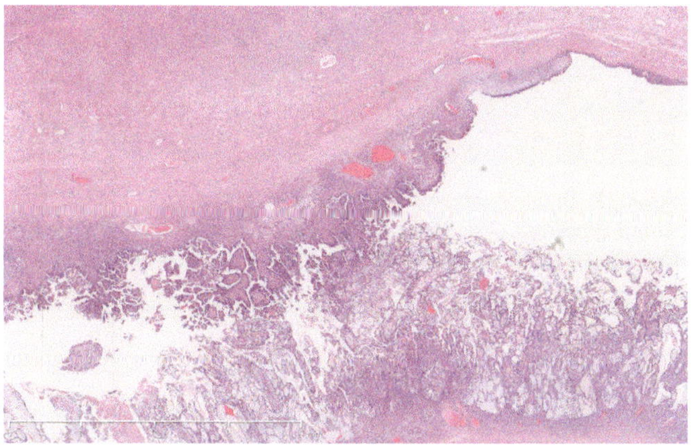

Fig. 4.20 Another example of direct continuity between endometriosis and a CCC, again arising within a cyst

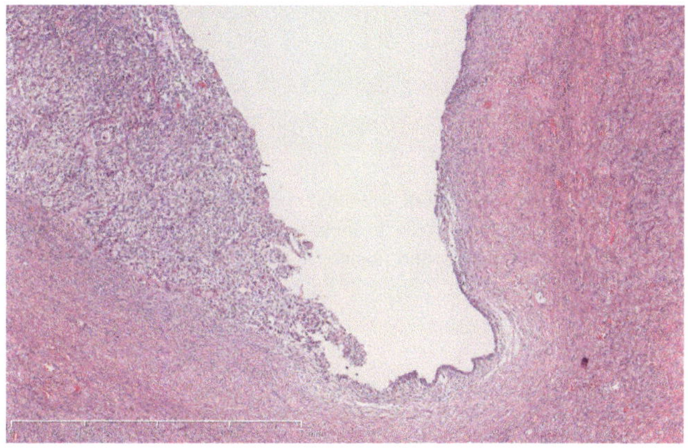

Fig. 4.21 Somewhat higher-power magnification of another case showing CCC arising in and from endometriosis

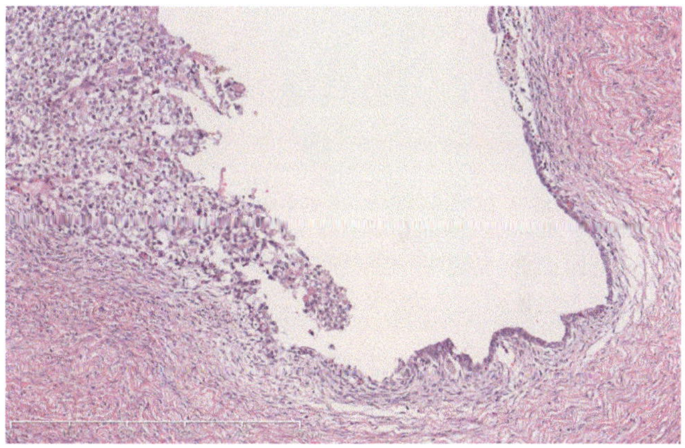

Fig. 4.22 In this figure, the presence of endometrial stroma beneath the benign-appearing endometrial epithelium of endometriosis is clearly seen, as is its absence beneath the CCC

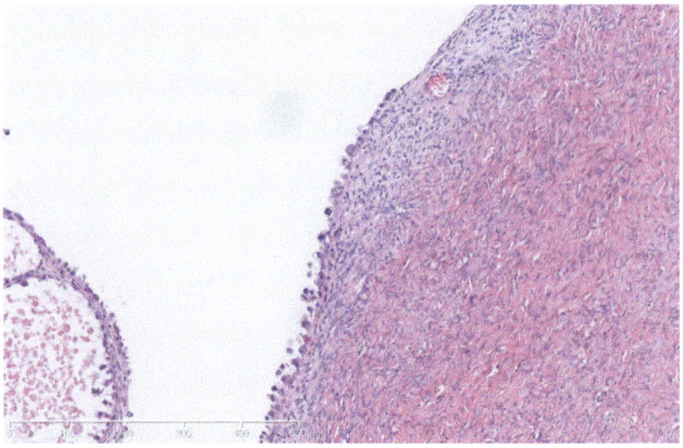

Fig. 4.23 In this illustration, the most common type of atypical endometriosis found in these cases is shown. The endometriosis is atypical by virtue of proliferation and nuclear atypia of the cells overlying the endometrioid stroma

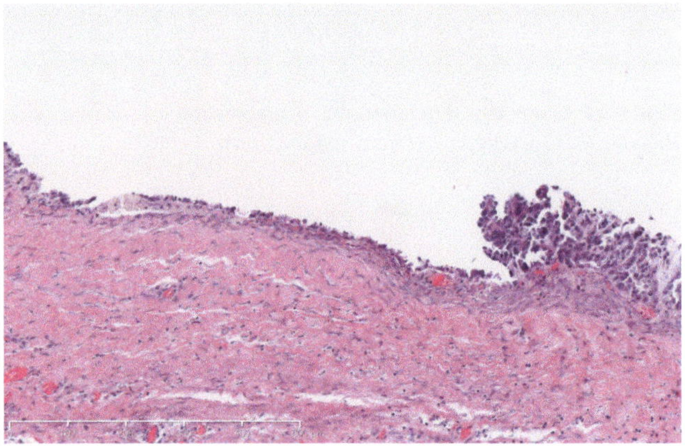

Fig. 4.24 Again, benign-appearing endometriosis leads into a focus resembling adenocarcinoma but still overlying endometrioid stroma. By convention, we diagnose this as atypical endometriosis

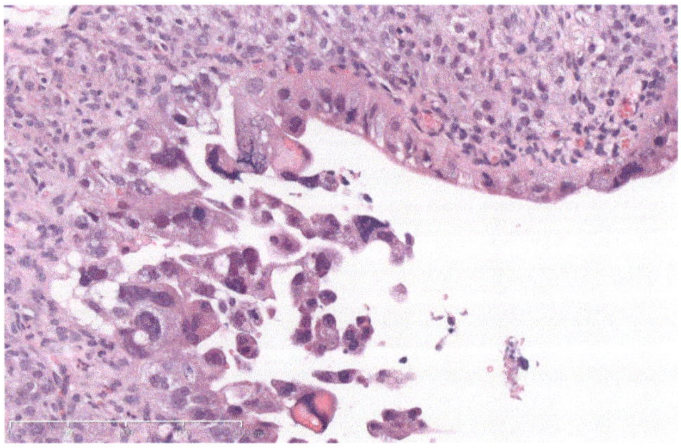

Fig. 4.25 A focus from another case showing non-atypical endometriosis leading into a field of atypical glandular proliferation, both with underlying endometrioid stroma. Again, this is diagnosable as atypical endometriosis and was contiguous with tumor

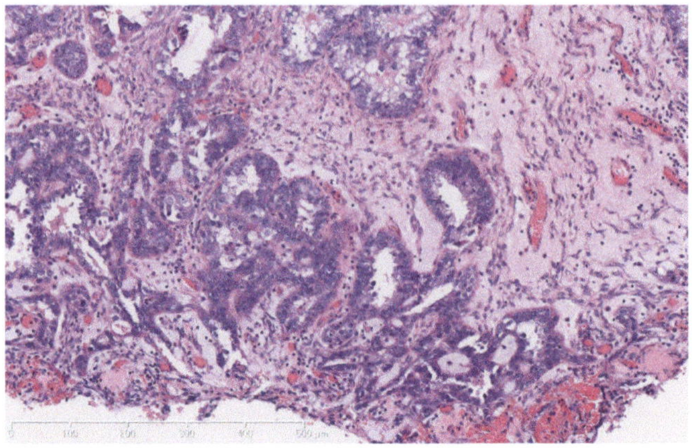

Fig. 4.26 This area of endometriosis is atypical by virtue of its glandular proliferation, resembling complex hyperplasia of the endometrium, rather than by virtue of nuclear atypia alone. This pattern of atypical endometriosis is less likely to be associated with CCC

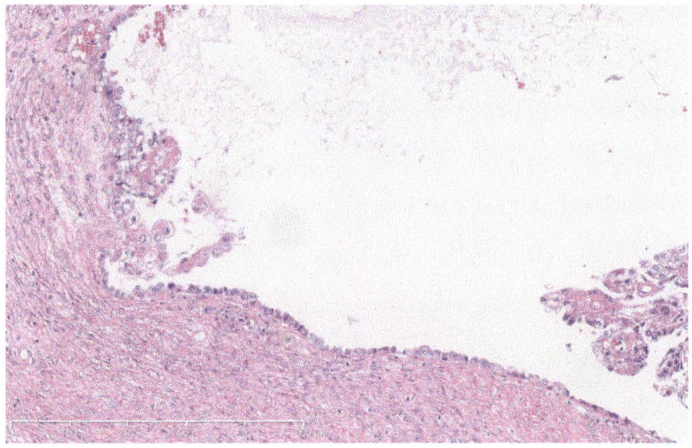

Fig. 4.27 In this figure, we see an ovarian CCC arising within a large benign-appearing cyst. However, no endometrial-type stroma is evident, so at least in this focus, the diagnosis of endometriosis cannot be made

Other histologic findings in ovarian CCC which are either less specific and/or less common than those mentioned above include stromal inflammatory infiltrates (Figs. 4.28, 4.29, and 4.30), often in tumor necrosis, occasionally with formation of cholesterol clefts (Figs. 4.31, 4.32, and 4.33), stromal fibrosis (Fig. 4.34), stromal edema (Fig. 4.35), pools of mucinous material in the stroma (Fig. 4.36), clefts around nests of tumor (Fig. 4.37), multinodularity (Figs. 4.38 and 4.39), thanatosomes [3] representing apoptotic tumor cells (Figs. 4.40 and 4.41), and foci of calcification, with occasional formation of psammoma bodies and rarely ossification (Figs. 4.42, 4.43, 4.44, 4.45, and 4.46).

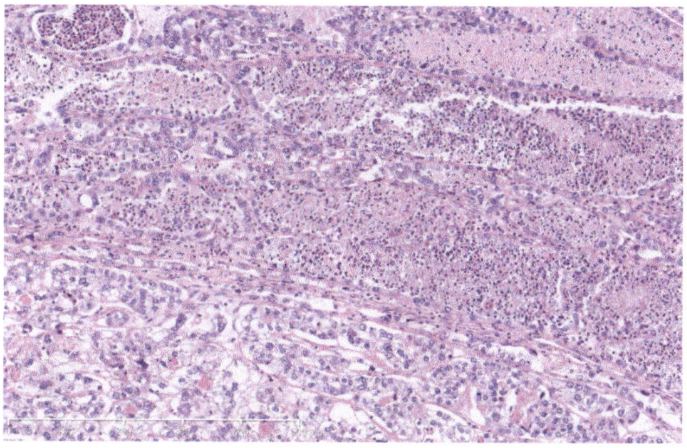

Fig. 4.28 Necro-inflammatory foci are occasionally seen in CCC, as illustrated here

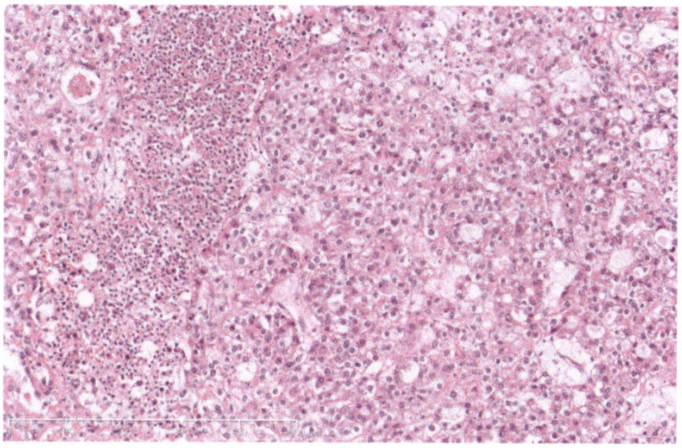

Fig. 4.30 In this field, the band of inflammatory cells between solid masses of tumor cells raises the differential diagnosis with dysgerminoma

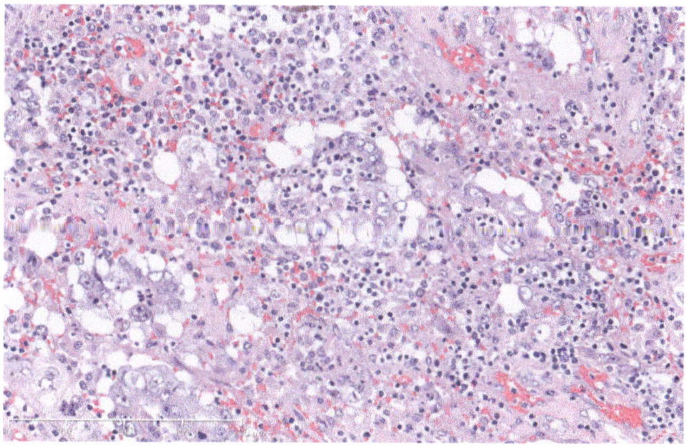

Fig. 4.29 A higher-power view of an inflammatory type of tumor necrosis

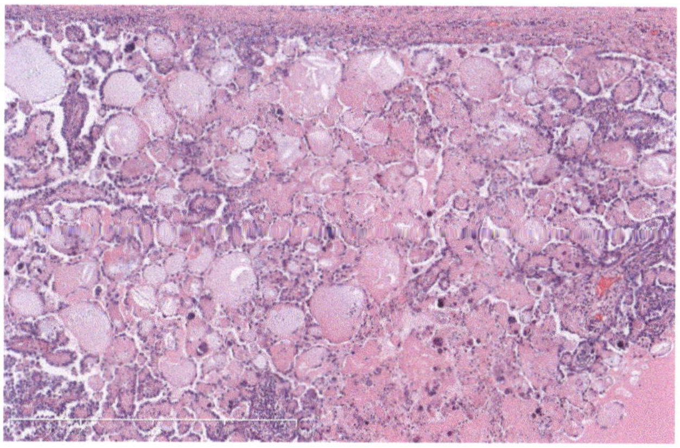

Fig. 4.31 As in any ovarian carcinoma, focal or extensive necrosis is common, as illustrated in this figure

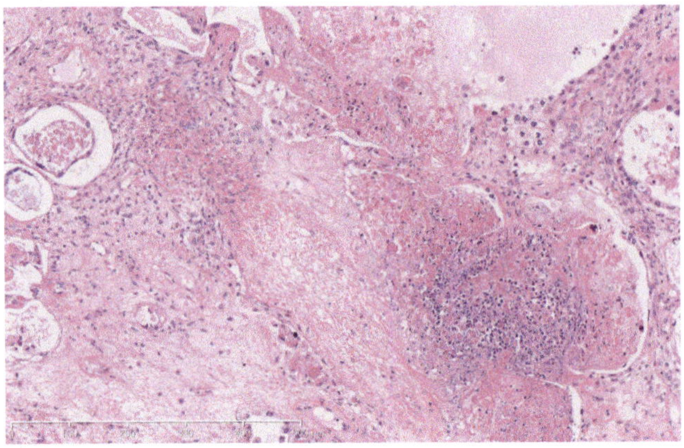

Fig. 4.32 Another large field of necrotic tumor. More viable tumor is not present, so it might be difficult to make the appropriate diagnosis

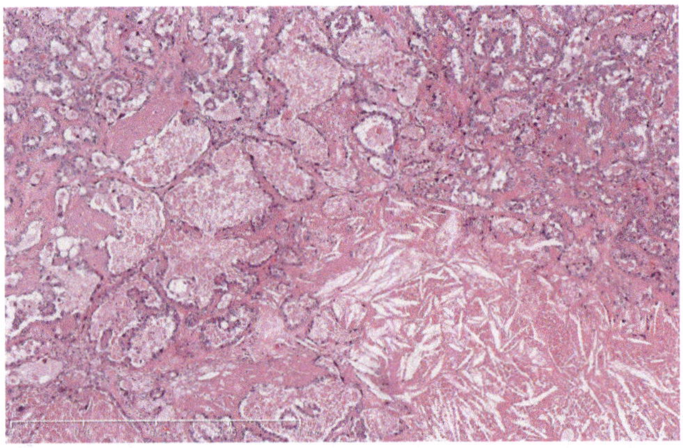

Fig. 4.33 Cholesterol clefts are occasionally found within CCC

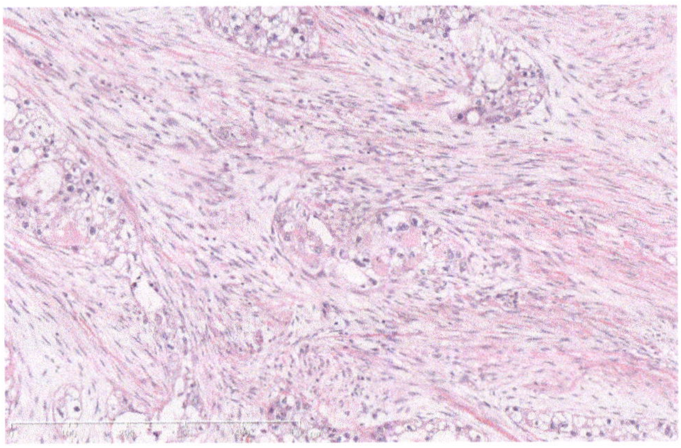

Fig. 4.34 True stromal fibrosis (other than that in the adenofibromatous pattern) is also rare in CCC

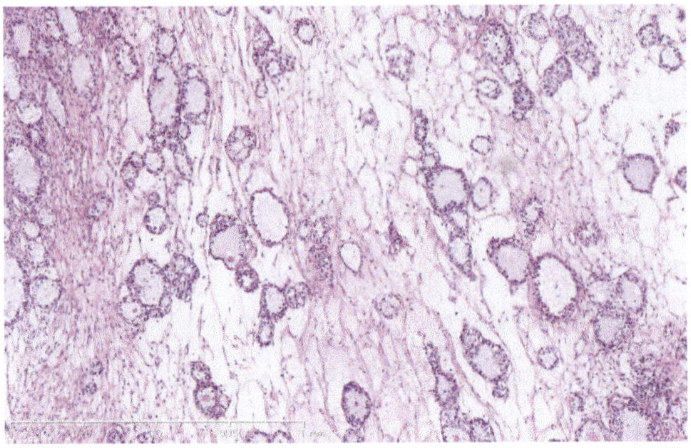

Fig. 4.35 Foci of stromal edema are rarely present, probably also indicating nearby necrosis

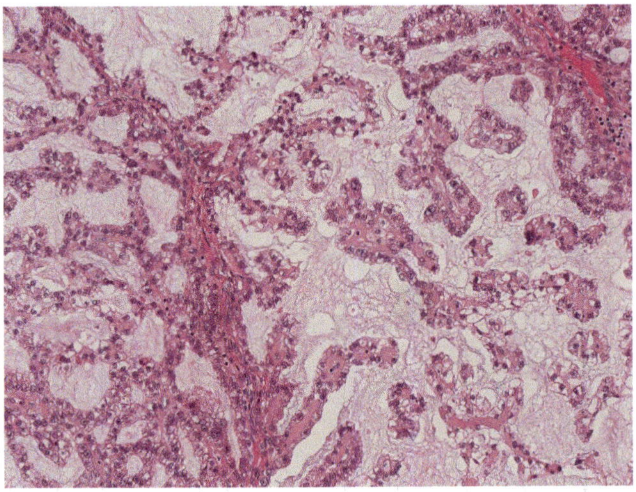

Fig. 4.36 Occasionally, large amounts of stromal mucinous material are present

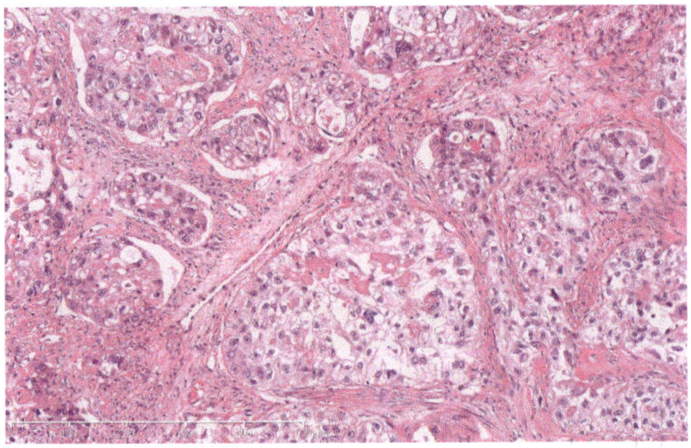

Fig. 4.37 In rare cases, clefts are noted around nests of tumor. It should be ascertained that these are not vascular spaces lined by endothelial cells, which would strongly favor a diagnosis of metastatic carcinoma to the ovary

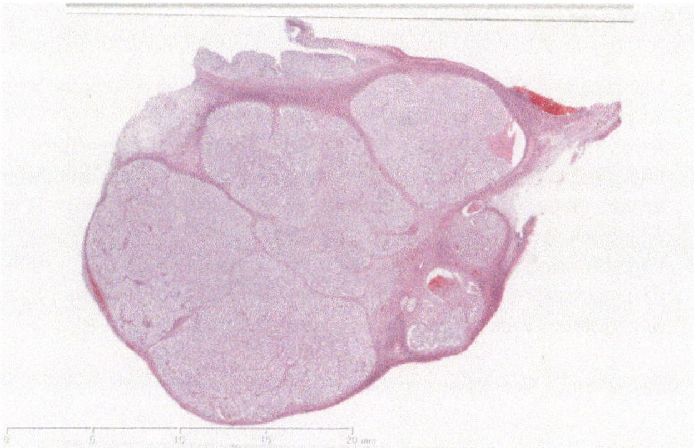

Fig. 4.38 Occasional tumors are noted to be multinodular. Again, this pattern might suggest a metastasis to the ovary, but in this case, endometriosis is also seen contiguous with the carcinoma

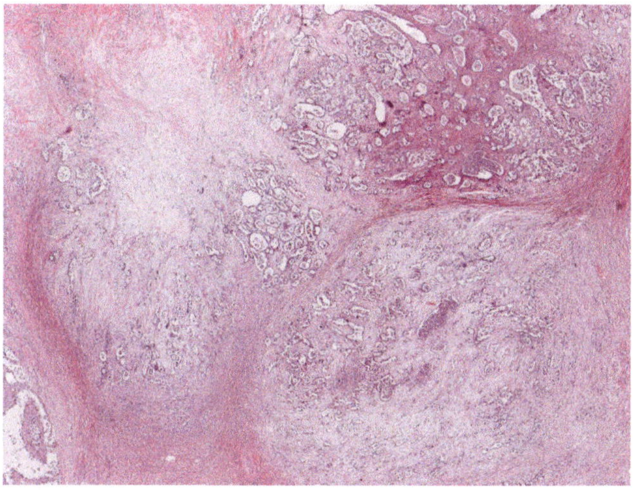

Fig. 4.39 Another multinodular pattern in ovarian CCC. The diagnosis of metastasis to the ovary was entertained, but other fields of this tumor were classical ovarian CCC

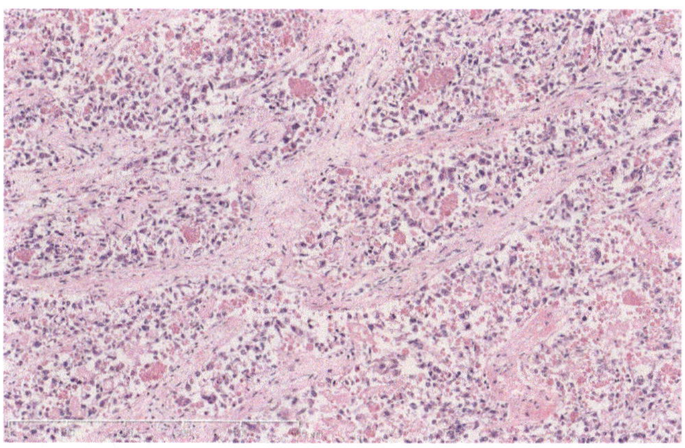

Fig. 4.40 This was our only case in which numerous thanatosomes were present. These represent apoptosis within tumor cells, as seen in the following figure

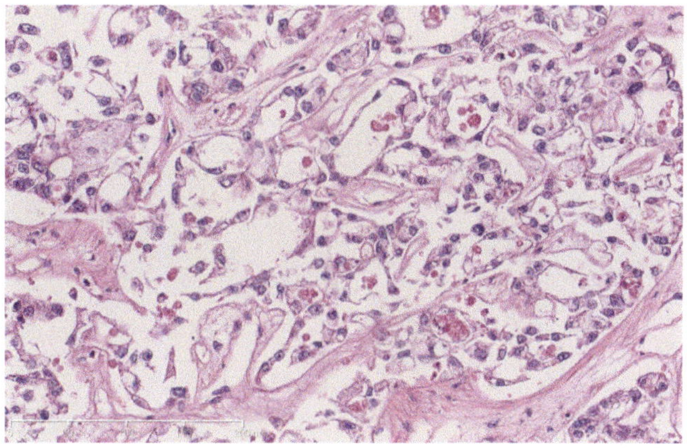

Fig. 4.41 More thanatosomes at higher power, seen in both intracellular and intercellular locations

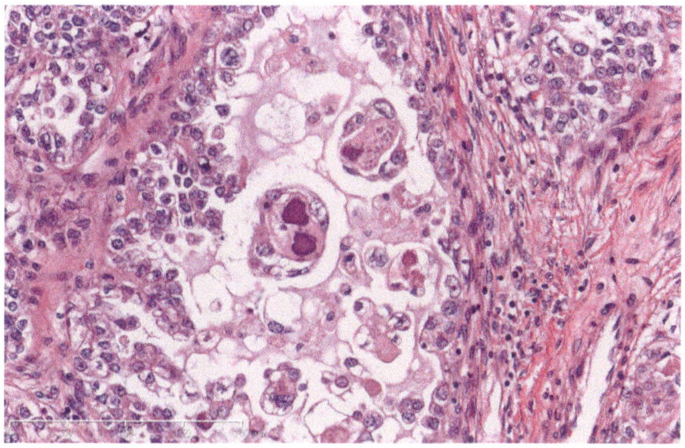

Fig. 4.42 Microcalcifications within tumor are a fairly common but totally nonspecific finding. This illustration shows a few early microcalcifications within an otherwise typical CCC

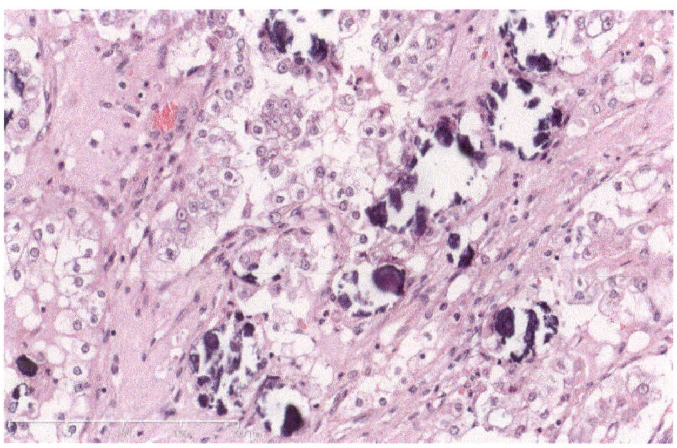

Fig. 4.43 In this tumor, microcalcifications are more frequent, and some of them form typical appearing psammoma bodies. The cellular background, however, is definitely that of a CCC rather than a serous carcinoma

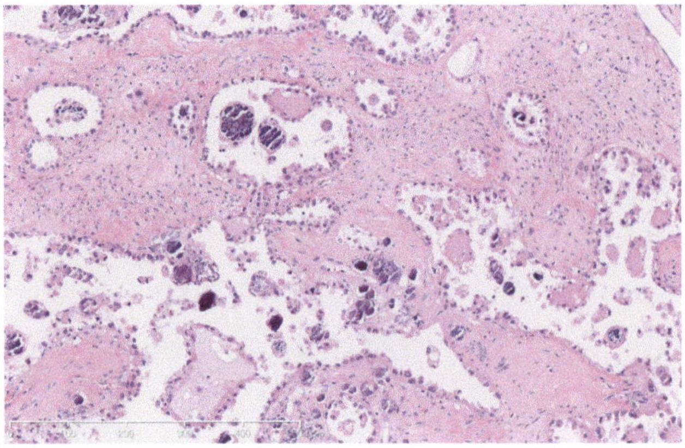

Fig. 4.44 Another case with extensive microcalcifications within the stroma of tumor micropapillae

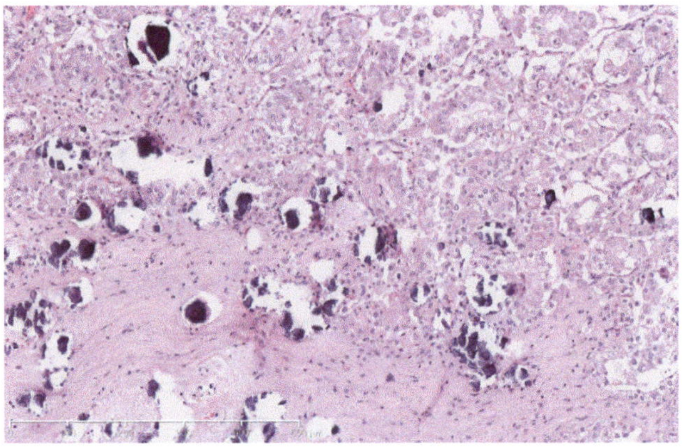

Fig. 4.45 In this field, extensive microcalcification has occurred, probably on the basis of preexisting necrosis and fibrosis

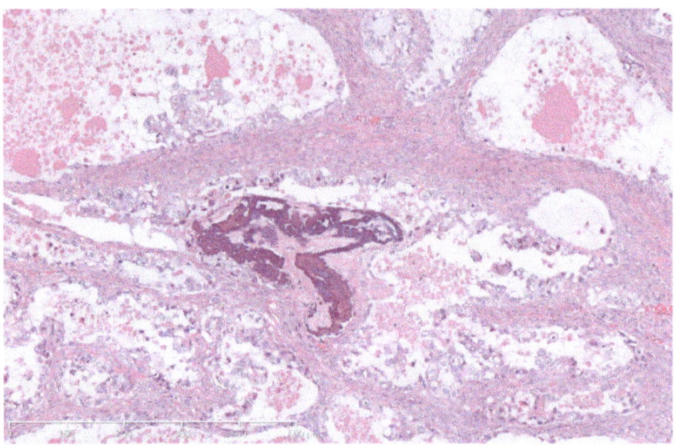

Fig. 4.46 In this tumor, some of the calcified foci have progressed to ossification. It should be noted that no malignant osteoblasts were identified, so this was not a carcinosarcoma of the ovary

References

1. LaGrenade A, Silverberg SG (1988) Ovarian tumors associated with atypical endometriosis. Hum Pathol 19:1080–1084
2. Veras E, Mao TL, Ayhan A et al (2009) Cystic and adenofibromatous clear cell carcinomas of the ovary: distinctive tumors that differ in their pathogenesis and behavior: a clinicopathologic analysis of 122 cases. Am J Surg Pathol 33:844–853
3. Papadimitriou JC, Drachenberg CB, Brenner DS et al (2000) "Thanatosomes". A unifying morphogenetic concept for tumor hyaline globules related to apoptosis. Hum Pathol 31:1455–1465

5 Histopathologic Grading

Grading of epithelial ovarian carcinomas has always been somewhat problematic, with different systems proposed for different histopathologic types [1]. Clear cell adenocarcinoma (CCC) has been the most problematic of all cell types, with almost all studies in the older literature failing to demonstrate a correlation between any grading system and survival (either disease-free or overall). This may have been, at least in part, because most published studies prior to the 1990s consisted of no more than 30 or 40 cases.

In 1998, Shimizu and colleagues [2, 3] proposed a "universal grading system" for ovarian epithelial carcinoma, which was meant to be applicable to all histopathologic types. In their own series, which consisted of over 400 cases overall, the system correlated well with survival for all cases, for early- and advanced-stage cases considered separately, and for all major cell types with the exception of CCC. The separation of survival of Grade 1, 2, and 3 cases according to the new system was statistically significant for all other cell types studied but only "suggestive" for CCC. Subsequent reports from other investigators have confirmed the applicability of this grading system to ovarian epithelial cancer in general but with variable results (usually similar to those of the Shimizu group) for CCC [4–6].

The most likely reason for the poorer results with CCC lies within the mechanics of the grading system itself and the usual histologic appearances of CCC. The system is based on assigning numerical scores for each of three microscopic features and then adding the scores for an individual tumor to determine the final grade. [1] Scores of 1–3 are assigned to each of the following features: (1) predominant architectural pattern (glandular/tubulocystic = 1, papillary = 2, solid = 3), (2) highest level of nuclear atypia (mild = 1, moderate = 2, severe = 3; these levels of atypia being defined more specifically in the Shimizu/Silverberg reports [1–3]), and (3) mitotic activity (0–9 mitotic figures counted per 10 high-power fields = 1, 10–25 MF/10 HPF = 2, 26 or more MF/10HPF = 3). When the three scores are added, a final tally of 3–5 is Grade 1, 6 or 7 is Grade 2, and 8 or 9 is Grade 3.

The problem with applying this system to CCC lies in the fact that CCC is always paucimitotic, so the score for mitotic activity will be 1 in the great majority of cases. Atypia is also not very variable, with most CCCs scoring 2 or 3 for nuclear atypia. Thus, the variability within a pool of CCC cases being graded is less than for most other epithelial ovarian carcinomas. We did not perform grading on all of the cases in the CCC series which form the basis for this Atlas, but at one point, we did grade a subset of these cases by the Shimizu system. Of 56 cases so graded, presumably representative of the entire series, 33 were Grade 1, 23 Grade 2, and none Grade 3. By individual scores, the mitotic score was 1 (fewer than 9 MF/10 HPF) in 52 of the 56 cases, with 3 cases scoring 2 and only one scoring 3 (and probably either the mitotic count or the diagnose of CCC is suspect in this case). Both nuclear atypia and architectural pattern peaked at scores of 2 (35 cases with this score for each of these determinations). A recent study of 129 graded CCC cases from Korea [7] reported similar findings but with a more uniform spread of architectural scores (38, 37, and 25 % scores 1, 2, and 3, respectively) and more skewing of nuclear atypia scores toward the severe level (57 % scoring 3 in this determination). As in our series, the majority of tumors (72.1 %) had a mitotic score of 1, with only 5.4 % scored as 3. Because of the higher estimation of nuclear atypia in this series, 52.7 % of cases received a universal grade of 2 or 3 (compared to 75.2 % FIGO Grade 2 or 3).

Citing these difficulties encountered in applying the Shimizu grading system to CCC, Yamamoto and colleagues [8] have subsequently proposed a new grading based on architectural features alone. Since the architectural patterns are the most variable from case to case, this would appear to be a reasonable approach if it were shown to be reproducible and to correlate with survival. As described by the authors, a tumor was assigned to Group A if it showed "entirely or mostly (more than or equal to 90 %) well-differentiated (or well-constructed) tubulocystic and/or papillary growth architecture..." and the proportion of less differentiated components was less than 10 %. These less differentiated

J. Kigawa et al., *Atlas of Clear Cell Carcinoma of the Ovary: A Pathological Guide*,
DOI 10.1007/978-4-431-55438-7_5, © Springer Japan 2015

components, present by definition for Group B in more than 10 % of a tumor, were described as "solid-appearing growth with fusiform glandular or papillary architecture" and "infiltrative small tubular pattern characterized by variously shaped, small glands of tumor cells." These so-called less differentiated components were distinguished from "very poorly differentiated components," which should be present in less than 10 % of a Group B tumor and more than 10 % of a Group C CCC. They were defined as "solid sheet-like tumor cell growth, or cord or diffuse infiltrative architecture with little or no glandular spaces." It was further stipulated that "small foci of glandular formations by tumor cells with their long axis perpendicular to the lumen may be discerned" in Group C tumors, "but should not exceed 1 distinct glandular space in a low-power field (5.51 mm^2 using 10× objective lens)." Although this may sound a bit difficult to reproduce, the reproducibility between two of the participating authors was excellent (no studies of reproducibility by nonparticipating pathologists have yet been reported). Survival at 5 years in this series of 159 patients was statistically significantly worse (15.4 %) in Group C compared with Groups A (51.1 %) and B (48.1 %), with Groups A and B not differing from one another.

In summary, it would appear that, at the present time, a tumor grading system for CCC that is both demonstrably reproducible outside the original investigative group and strongly related to survival in both low- and high-stage cases cannot be shown to exist. The most recent (2014) World Health Organization (WHO) publication on ovarian tumors [9] states that "…the nuclear grade is nearly always high regardless of the grading system used, and for that reason all clear cell carcinomas are considered high grade." Despite the fact that this WHO manual agrees that mitotic activity "tends to be low," this is the most recent and probably the most accurate statement on CCC grading at the present time.

References

1. Silverberg SG (2000) Histopathologic grading of ovarian carcinoma: a review and proposal. Int J Gynecol Pathol 19:7–15
2. Shimizu Y, Kamoi S, Amada S, Hasumi K et al (1998) Toward the development of a universal grading system for ovarian epithelial carcinoma: 1. Prognostic significance of histopathologic features – problems involved in the architectural grading system. Gynecol Oncol 70:2–12
3. Shimizu Y, Kamoi S, Amada S et al (1998) Toward the development of a universal grading system for ovarian epithelial carcinoma: testing of a proposed system in a series of 461 patients with uniform treatment and follow-up. Cancer 82:893–901
4. Ishioka S, Sagae S, Terasawa K et al (2000) Comparison of the usefulness between a new universal grading system for epithelial ovarian cancer and the FIGO grading system. Gynecol Oncol 89:447–452
5. Ryu SY, Park SI, Nam BH et al (2009) Prognostic significance of histologic grade in clear-cell carcinoma of the ovary: a retrospective study of Korean Gynecologic Oncology Group. Ann Oncol 20:1032–1036
6. Yamamoto S, Kasajima A, Takano M et al (2011) Validation of the histological grading for ovarian clear cell carcinoma: a retrospective multi-institutional study by the Japan Clear Cell Carcinoma Study Group. Int J Gynecol Pathol 30:129–138
7. Min K-W, Park MH, Hong SR, Lee H et al (2013) Clear cell carcinomas of the ovary: a multi-institutional study Of 129 cases in Korea with prognostic significance of Emi1 and Galactin-3. Int J Gynecol Pathol 32:3–14
8. Yamamoto S, Tsuda H, Shimazaki H et al (2012) histological grading of ovarian clear cell carcinoma: proposal for a simple and reproducible grouping system based on tumor growth architecture. Int J Gynecol Pathol 31:116–124
9. Kurman RJ, Carcangiu ML, Herringyon CS, Young RH (eds) (2014) WHO classification of tumours of female reproductive organs. International Agency for Research on Cancer, Lyon

6 Immunohistochemistry

The immunohistochemical literature on ovarian clear cell carcinoma (CCC) is, like many other subjects, hampered by both small series of reported cases and the use of "house pet" antibodies which are generally unavailable in the outside world. Although our own series which forms the basis of this Atlas consists of more than 600 cases, the material available for centralized pathologic review consisted almost exclusively of hematoxylin- and eosin (H&E)-stained slides, so this chapter will consist predominantly of a brief review of the diagnostically and/or prognostically significant literature.

CCC shares with other ovarian epithelial carcinomas diffuse strong immunoreactivity for epithelial markers including CK7, CAM5.2, and EMA. These can occasionally be useful in the differential diagnosis with non-epithelial tumors featuring clear or oxyphil/oncocytic cells, but are not helpful in the distinction of CCC from primary ovarian serous, endometrioid, and mutinous carcinomas [1].

On the other hand, there is a subset of antibodies that has been found useful in these distinctions (Figs. 6.1 and 6.2) [1–4]. In a study of interobserver reproducibility in the diagnosis of ovarian carcinoma histotype, Kobel and colleagues [1] found a high level of interobserver agreement with the use of H&E slides alone but also noted significant improvement when an immunohistochemical panel consisting of WT-1, p53, p16, HNF-1 beta, ARID1A, and progesterone receptor (PR) was added to the review. Others have also confirmed these observations, particularly for CCC. In a study of 155 cases, DeLair and colleagues characterized the immunoprofile of CCC as HNF positive and ER/PR/WT-1/p53 negative [2]. As the only consistently positive marker for CCC in this group, HNF-1 beta (hepatocyte nuclear factor-1 beta) is particularly valuable. In one study [3], 21 of 22 CCC and only one of 61 non-CCC ovarian cancer specimens were found to have strong nuclear staining for this marker; the authors also confirmed upregulation of HNF-1 beta in CCC by real-time quantitative reverse transcription-polymerase chain reaction and immunoblotting and suggested HNF-1beta as a possible molecular target for CCC therapy.

J. Kigawa et al., *Atlas of Clear Cell Carcinoma of the Ovary: A Pathological Guide*,
DOI 10.1007/978-4-431-55438-7_6, © Springer Japan 2015

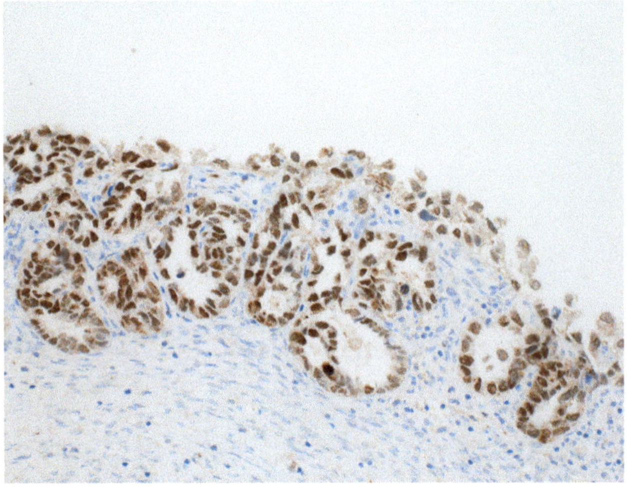

Fig. 6.1 Strongly positive HNF-1beta nuclear immunostaining in a clear cell carcinoma

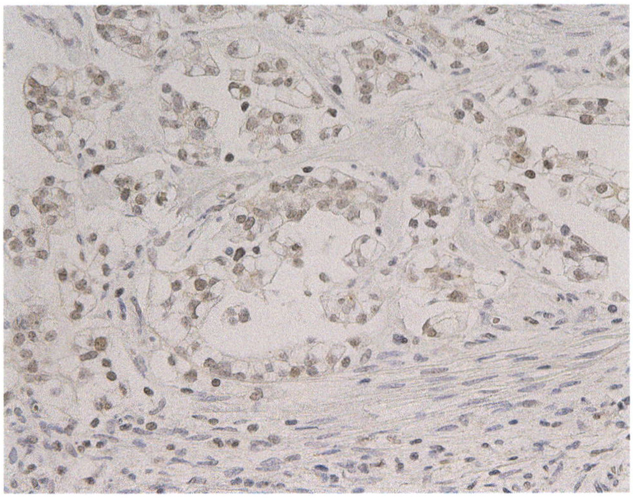

Fig. 6.2 Diffuse moderate nuclear reactivity for ARID1A in a clear cell carcinoma. Note: sections of 4-mm thickness were cut from the paraffin blocks of CCC. Each section was mounted on a glass slide, deparaffinized, and soaked in 0.3 % H_2O_2/methanol for 15 min at room temperature to block endogenous peroxidase. HNF-1beta staining: the slides were pretreated with EnVision™ FLEX Target Retrieval Solution, High pH (1:50) (DAKO) using PT-Link system (DAKO) for heat-induced epitope retrieval at 97 °C for 20 min. After blocking intrinsic peroxidases with 0.1 % H_2O_2, the slides were incubated with the goat antihuman HNF polyclonal antibody (C-20: Santa Cruz, sc-7411) (1:2,000) at 4 °C for 17 h. After washing out the extra primary antibodies by several rinses in PBS, the slides were incubated with the secondary antibody (rabbit anti-goat immunoglobulins (DAKO), 1:200) at room temperature for 30 min. The location of HNF-1beta on the slides was visualized with DAB after adding EnVision™ FLEX+Rabbit (LINKER) (DAKO). ARID1A: a mouse monoclonal anti-ARID1A (1:500; Santa Cruz Biotechnology, Santa Cruz, CA) was applied for 2 h at 37 °C. The primary antibody was visualized using the Histofine Simple Stain PO (M) kit (Nichirei, Tokyo, Japan) according to the instruction manual. The slide was counterstained with hematoxylin

WT-1 has proven to be a useful immunomarker for the distinction of CCC from serous carcinoma of the ovary (serous carcinomas 90 % or more positive vs. around 20 % of CCCs) [4]. Since endometrioid and mucinous carcinomas, as well as many other primary and metastatic ovarian tumors, are also WT-1 negative, serous carcinoma is the only mimic of CCC ruled out by WT-1 negativity, and even this is not absolute.

The story is similar for estrogen (ER) and progesterone (PR) receptors. One of the largest studies reported to date [5] noted that 81 % of 381 CCCs examined for ER immunoreactivity were negative and 92 % of 363 studied cases were PR negative. High-grade serous, low-grade serous, and endometrioid carcinomas were all more likely to be strongly immunoreactive for ER (60, 71, and 60 %, respectively), but PR status was less reliable as a distinguishing marker, since 69, 43, and 33 %, respectively, of these tumors were PR negative. Mucinous carcinomas, like CCCs, were usually negative for both ER (70 %) and PR (84 %). Furthermore, a small proportion of CCCs were strongly immunoreactive for ER (14 %) and/or PR (3 %).

p53 is also a useful marker in only a small proportion of cases and for CCC is another negative marker; its major efficacy is in the differential diagnosis with high-grade serous carcinoma, which almost always has TP53 overexpression [1]. ARID1A protein loss of expression may be limited to CCC and endometrioid carcinoma among major ovarian cancers, but this is still neither well proven nor widely available [1].

A few other markers have recently been recommended for predictive or prognostic purposes. Low proliferative activity as measured by Ki-67 labeling has been reported as a possible association with chemoresistance in CCC, with the labeling index being significantly higher in responders than nonresponders; whether this is independent of mitotic counting is not yet known [6]. The same group of investigators also reported that galactin-3 expression was common (70 %) in CCC and might contribute to chemoresistance [7]. A recent report [8] has suggested that CXCR4 high immunoexpression in CCC was associated with poorer overall and progression-free survival, but this observation is awaiting confirmation before wide usage of this antibody is recommended.

References

1. Kobel M, Bak J, Bertelsen BI, Carpen O et al (2014) Ovarian carcinoma histotype determination if highly reproducible, and is improved through the use of immunohistochemistry. Histopathology 64:1004–1013. doi:10.1111/his 12349
2. DeLair D, Oliva E, Kobel M, Macias A et al (2011) Morphologic spectrum of immunohistochemically characterized clear cell carcinoma of the ovary: a study of 155 cases. Am J Surg Pathol 35:36–44
3. Tsuchiya A, Sakamoto M, Yasuda J, Chuma M et al (2003) Expression profiling in ovarian clear cell carcinoma: identification of hapatocyte nuclear factor-1 beta as a molecular marker and a possible molecular target for therapy of ovarian clear cell carcinoma. Am J Pathol 163:2503–2512
4. Acs G, Pasha T, Zhang PJ (2004) WT1 is differentially expressed in serous, endometrioid, clear cell, and mutinous carcinomas of the peritoneum, fallopian tube, ovary, and endometrium. Int J Gynecol Pathol 23:110–118
5. Sieh W, Kobel M, Longacre TA, Bowtell DD et al (2013) Hormone-receptor expression and ovarian cancer survival: an Ovarian Tumor Tissue Analysis consortium study. Lancet Oncol 14:853–862
6. Itamochi H, Kigawa J, Sugiyama T et al (2002) Low proliferation activity may be associated with chemoresistance in clear cell carcinoma of the ovary. Obstet Gynecol 100:281–287
7. Oishi T, Itamochi H, Kigawa J et al (2007) Galectin-3 may contribute to Cisplatin resistance in clear cell carcinoma of the ovary. Int J Gynecol Cancer 17:1040–1046
8. Sekiya R, Kajiyama H, Sakai K et al (2012) Expression of CXCR4 indicates poor prognosis in patients with clear cell carcinoma of the ovary. Hum Pathol 43:904–910

7 Differential Diagnosis

As mentioned earlier in this volume, a very small number of the more than 600 cases submitted to our study as clear cell carcinoma (CCC) of the ovary were rejected for inappropriate histopathologic documentation, suggesting that the differential diagnosis of CCC is not a major cause of concern for most diagnostic pathologists. Of course, we have no way of knowing how many cases were not submitted because they were incorrectly diagnosed as something else, but we suspect that (at least in Japan, where CCC is a fairly common ovarian tumor and the index of suspicion is therefore high) not many cases were missed in this manner. In other countries where high-grade serous carcinoma may be ten times more common than CCC, the tendency certainly might be for an indeterminate case to be assigned to the serous rather than the clear cell category or to be called "mixed serous and clear cell" type, a term that is no longer recommended [1].

From a review in both of our own cases and of the literature, the differential diagnosis of ovarian CCC is predominantly with (in no particular order) (1) benign and borderline clear cell tumors; (2) other primary ovarian epithelial tumors, mainly carcinomas but occasionally borderline tumors; (3) ovarian germ cell and sex cord-stromal tumors; and (4) metastatic tumors in the ovary. These will be discussed in the order listed.

Although we have chosen to list and discuss benign and borderline clear cell tumors first, it is certainly not because these are either particularly common or particularly problematic. In fact, the current World Health Organization (WHO) Classification of Tumours of Female Reproductive Organs states that clear cell cystadenoma and adenofibroma "are very rare tumors, with only a few cases reported in the literature" and that clear cell borderline tumors "comprise less than 1 % of borderline/atypical proliferative tumours" [2]. We believe that clear cell borderline tumors are even rarer than benign clear cell tumors, perhaps because we use the term "atypical clear cell cystadenoma/adenofibroma" for noninvasive clear cell tumors with focal or diffuse cytologic atypia only (Fig. 7.1). In any event, the important fact to remember is that benign-appearing clear cell tumor foci with or without (Fig. 7.2) atypia are seen frequently within CCC; it is not known whether in this situation these foci are biologically benign or malignant. On the other hand, when an ovarian tumor consists exclusively of clear cell cystadenoma, adenofibroma, or borderline tumor on initial sections, it is certainly recommended to submit additional sections to rule out CCC manifested by stromal invasion.

J. Kigawa et al., *Atlas of Clear Cell Carcinoma of the Ovary: A Pathological Guide*,
DOI 10.1007/978-4-431-55438-7_7, © Springer Japan 2015

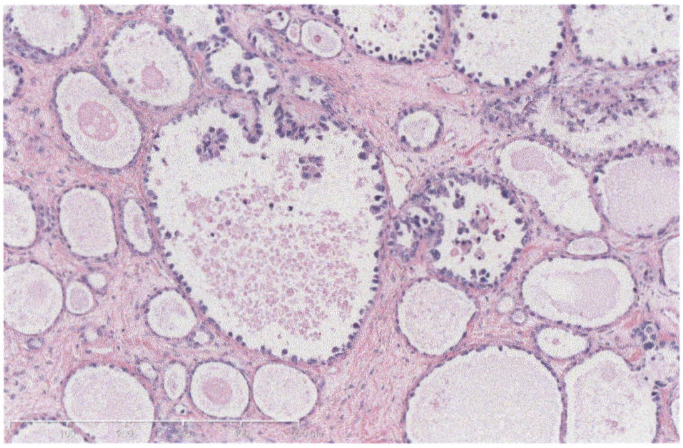

Fig. 7.1 Atypical clear cell adenofibroma focus within a clear cell adenocarcinoma. Some of the cystic glandular spaces are lined by hobnail cells with large atypical nuclei, some of which form cellular micropapillary projections within lumina. There is no evidence of stromal invasion

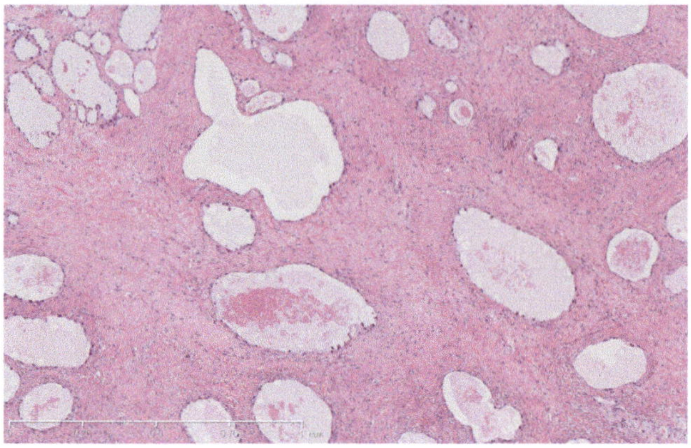

Fig. 7.2 Clear cell adenofibroma without atypia, also found as a focus within a clear cell carcinoma (CCC)

A much more common differential diagnostic problem is the distinction of CCC from other ovarian epithelial tumors, particularly high-grade serous carcinoma, endometrioid carcinoma, and serous borderline tumor. As mentioned above, when an ovarian carcinoma appears to contain areas of both serous and clear cell type, it is currently considered appropriate to classify this as a serous carcinoma [1]. A few legitimate CCCs in our series, on the other hand, did contain foci which superficially resembled serous borderline tumor (Fig. 7.3). Closer examination revealed that at higher magnification, the papillary structures were lined by the usual clear and hobnail cells and hyalinization of the stroma within the papillae was also typical for CCC. Endometrioid carcinoma was a more frequent cause of exclusion from our CCC series. These two carcinomas both often originate in endometriosis and often occur together as mixed carcinomas. We allowed small amounts of endometrioid carcinoma in a clear cell carcinoma but excluded those cases with major endometrioid components. In some excluded cases, the main problem was different initial and review assessments of the relative proportions of these two elements, but in others, it appeared that secretory endometrioid foci (Fig. 7.4) or squamous components with clear cytoplasm (Fig. 7.5) had been misinterpreted as CCC. It is important to search carefully for typical areas of CCC or of endometrioid carcinoma (Fig. 7.6) within such tumors in order to make the correct diagnosis.

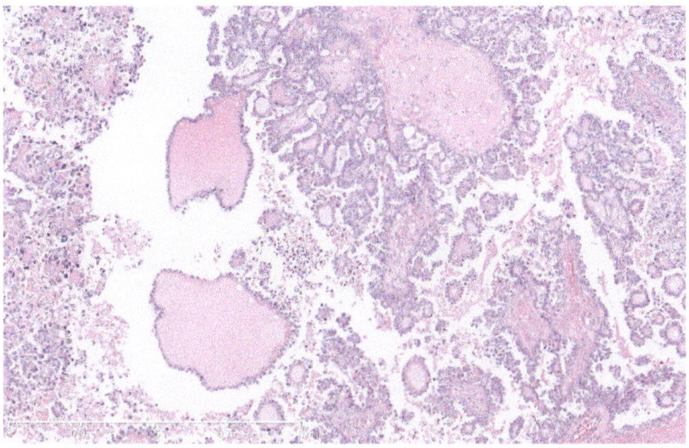

Fig. 7.3 Region within an otherwise typical CCC which resembled serous borderline tumor at low magnification, as seen here. Prominent stromal hyalinization seen here, as well as clear and hobnail cell lining of the micropapillae (better noted at higher magnification), indicates that this is a growth pattern of this CCC

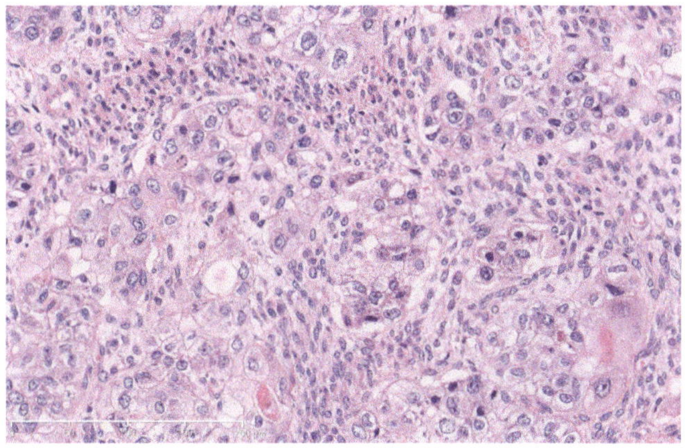

Fig. 7.5 Squamous differentiation within an endometrioid carcinoma. Clear cytoplasm within these squamous cells led to misclassification as CCC

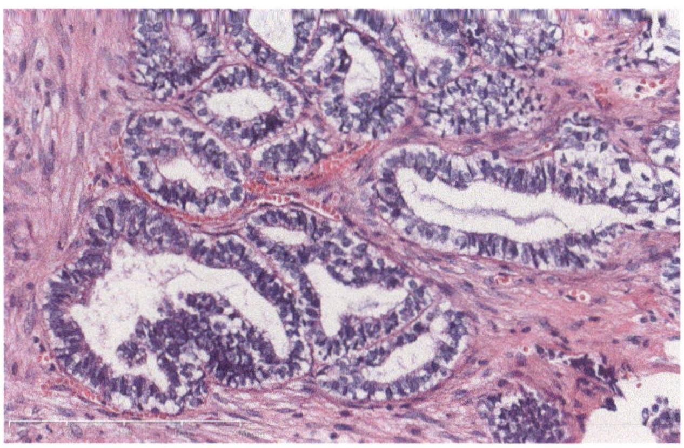

Fig. 7.4 Endometrioid carcinoma of secretory type. Subnuclear clear secretory vacuoles led to confusion with CCC

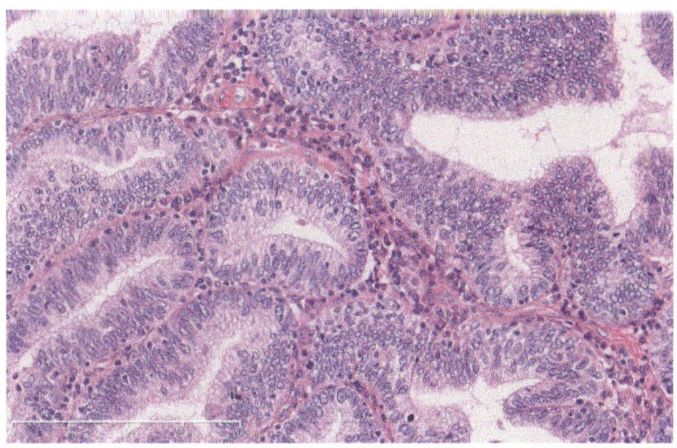

Fig. 7.6 More classical appearance of endometrioid carcinoma. Glands are lined by pseudostratified cuboidal to columnar epithelium in which the uniform small ovoid nuclei are lined up parallel to one another and perpendicular to the basement membrane

As discussed in more detail in Chap. 6 of this volume, immunohistochemistry can be helpful in certain difficult differential diagnostic problems [3]. HNF-1beta immunoreactivity is present in most CCCs, but not in serous or endometrioid carcinomas. On the other hand, CCC is typically negative for WT-1 (positive in most serous carcinomas) and progesterone receptor (PR, typically present in endometrioid carcinomas). Although the finding of endometriosis adjacent to a tumor is common in both CCC and endometrioid carcinoma, it is rare (2 % or less) in serous carcinoma, so this can be a useful diagnostic tool as well [4].

The differential diagnosis of CCC with primary ovarian tumors of non-epithelial type can be quite difficult on morphologic grounds alone, so clinical features and immunohistochemical findings are quite helpful. Germ cell tumors such as dysgerminoma (Figs. 7.7, 7.8, and 7.9) and yolk sac (endodermal sinus) tumor (Figs. 7.10, 7.11, 7.12, and 7.13) can be particularly problematic, so it is worth remembering that the youngest of our more than 600 CCC patients was 30 years old and most patients were 50 or above, whereas both yolk sac tumors and dysgerminomas occur predominantly between the ages of 15 and 25. Contiguous endometriosis is also rare in malignant germ cell tumors, and although particular microscopic fields may be vexing, examination of the entire sampled tumor will usually reveal classical CCC or one of its mimics. When immunohistochemical help is needed, positivity in CCC for epithelial markers such as cytokeratins will quickly rule out dysgerminoma, while yolk sac tumors are immunoreactive for alpha-fetoprotein (AFP) and SALL4 [5].

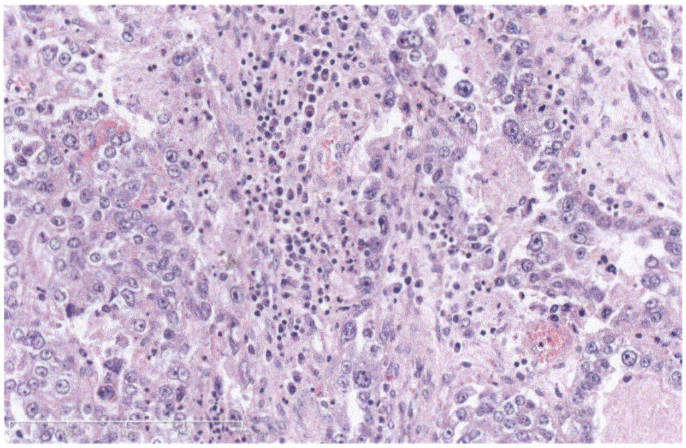

Fig. 7.7 Medium-power microscopic field within a CCC in which tumor cell nests separated by stroma rich in lymphocytes and plasma cells mimic the appearance of dysgerminoma

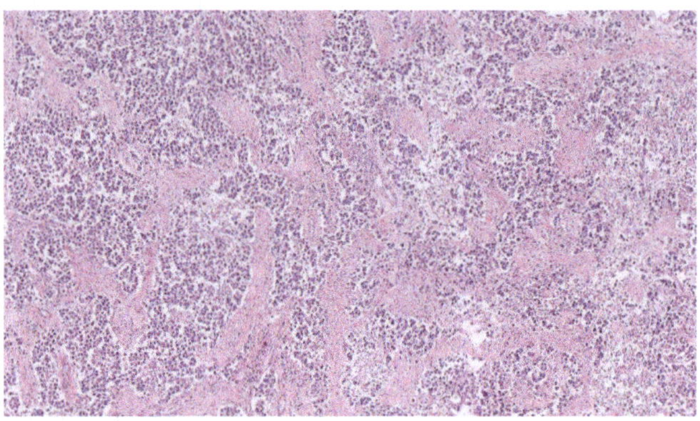

Fig. 7.8 True dysgerminoma with desmoplastic (but not hyalinized) stroma containing relatively few lymphocytes

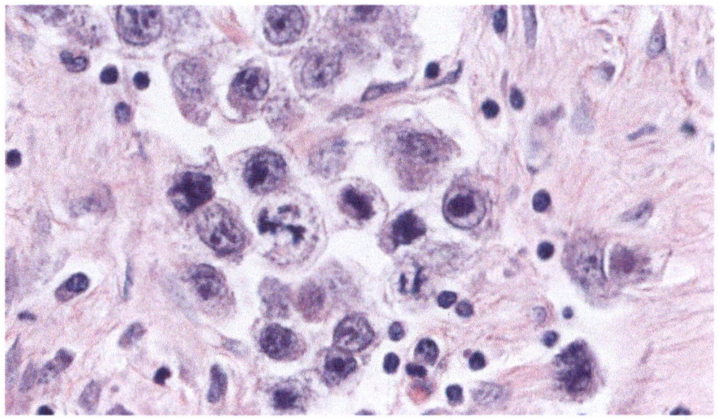

Fig. 7.9 High-power field of dysgerminoma includes some cells with clear cytoplasm. Unlike CCC, numerous mitotic figures are also encountered. Tubulocystic and papillary tumor growth are vanishingly rare in dysgerminoma but present at least focally in most CCCs

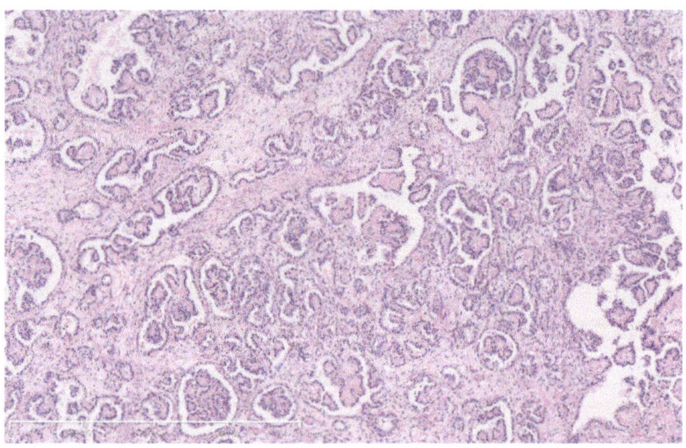

Fig. 7.10 CCC with micropapillae projecting into tubules, recalling the Schiller-Duval bodies seen in yolk sac (endodermal sinus) tumor. An unusually desmoplastic stroma is also present in this field, but elsewhere the tumor was typical CCC

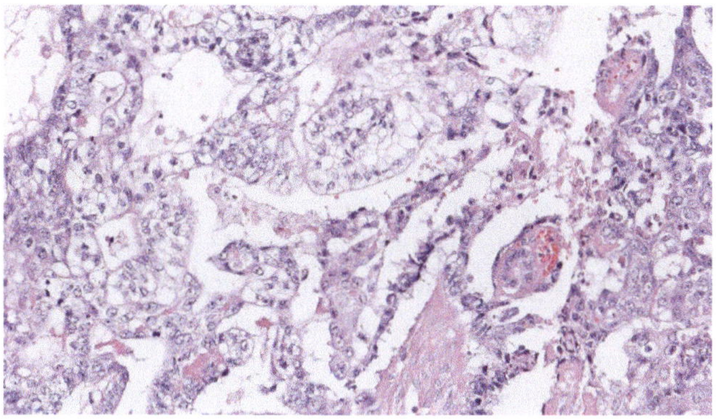

Fig. 7.11 True yolk sac tumor in a young patient. Note classical Schiller-Duval bodies and prominent clear cells

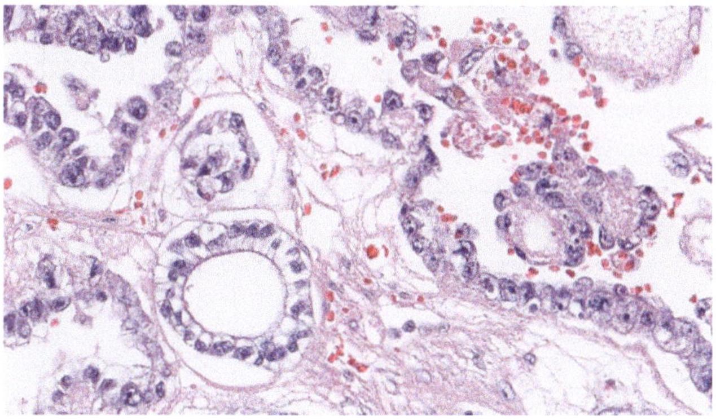

Fig. 7.12 Another field of yolk sac tumor, with both clear and oxyphilic cells

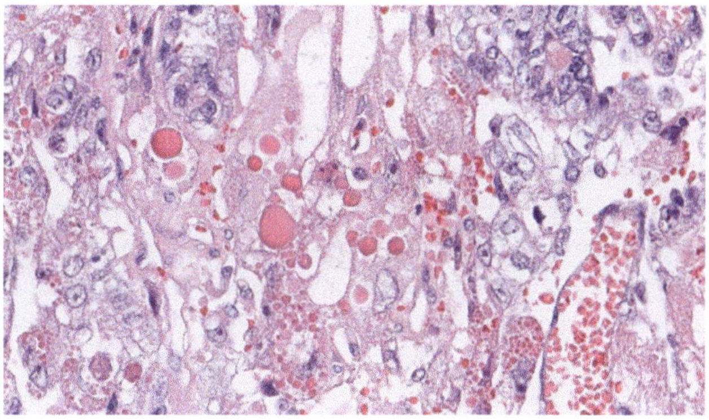

Fig. 7.13 Same yolk sac tumor as illustrated in Figs. 7.11 and 7.12. Numerous intra- and extracellular hyaline globules are present. These stain with PAS and alpha-fetoprotein immunostain and are classical for yolk sac tumor

Other primary ovarian non-epithelial tumors which can enter into the differential diagnosis of CCC on the basis of the presence of neoplastic cells with clear cytoplasm include steroid cell tumor, microcystic stromal tumor, and either struma ovarii or a sebaceous tumor arising as a monodermal teratoma. None of these has raised serious concerns in our experience. CCC with oxyphilic/oncocytic rather than clear cytoplasm can raise a somewhat different set of differential diagnostic possibilities, including Leydig cell tumor and hepatoid carcinoma; again, we have not seen these as serious diagnostic problems.

Finally, the differential diagnosis of CCC with metastatic tumors within the ovary can be a real problem and accounted for a high percentage of the cases rejected from our series. Metastatic renal cell carcinoma has been commented on most frequently in the literature [6], but an informal survey of prominent gynecologic pathologists by one of us (SGS) has not uncovered a single case of this diagnosis in surgical as opposed to autopsy material. Furthermore, except for the presence of clear cells, renal carcinomas look quite different from ovarian CCC, particularly in respect to their microvascular pattern, so immunohistochemical markers are not likely to be needed for this distinction. On the other hand, we did see cases in our series of metastases from other adenocarcinomas, particularly gastrointestinal, which were mistakenly submitted as primary ovarian CCC (Fig. 7.14). Although some of these had variable amounts of clear (or oxyphilic) cytoplasm, they were generally not difficult to distinguish from CCC by the usual criteria for metastases to the ovary (multinodularity, vascular invasion, prominent surface involvement, desmoplastic stroma, etc.) [7]. If doubt remains, immunohistochemical markers are usually helpful. Other metastases to the ovary which may be confused with CCC include thyroid and hepatic carcinomas and melanomas. Not mentioned prominently in the literature, and not encountered in our series (or at least not recognized by us), but potentially a cause of confusion, is metastatic CCC of endometrial or endocervical origin; the mimicry of primary ovarian CCC would presumably be even more deceptive in such cases, and the decision as to the primary lesion would be difficult at best.

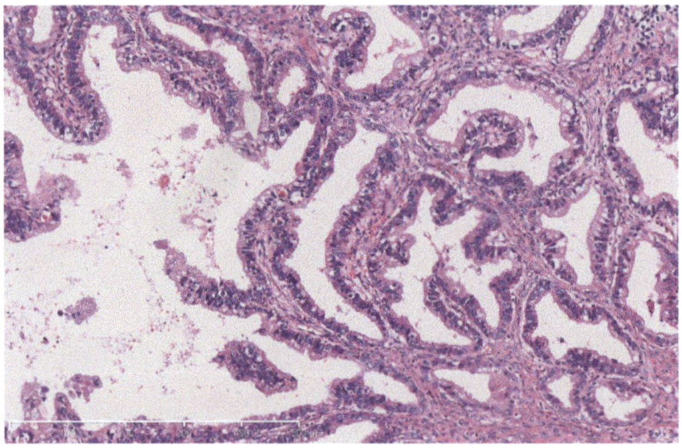

Fig. 7.14 Metastatic colorectal adenocarcinoma in ovary. It is difficult in retrospect to be sure why this tumor was submitted as CCC, but it and others like it were. This represents a significant problem in differential diagnosis (cf. text and Ref. [7])

References

1. Han G, Gilks CB, Leung S et al (2008) Mixed ovarian epithelial carcinomas with clear cell and serous components are variants of high-grade serous carcinoma: an interobserver correlative and immunohistochemical study of 32 cases. Am J Surg Pathol 32:955–964
2. Gilks CB, Bell DA, Huntsman D, Longacre TA et al (2014) Clear cell tumours. In: Kurman RJ, Carcangiu ML, Herrington CS, Young RH (eds) WHO classification of tumours of female reproductive organs. International Agency for Research on Cancer, Lyon, pp 33–35
3. Kobel M, Bak J, Bertelsen BI, Carpen O et al (2014) Ovarian carcinoma histotype is highly reproducible, and is improved through the use of immunohistochemistry. Histopathology 64:1004–1013. doi:10.1111/his.12349
4. Ogawa S, Kaku T, Amada S, Kobayashi H et al (2000) Ovarian endometriosis associated with ovarian carcinoma: a clinical and immunohistochemical study. Gynecol Oncol 77:298–304
5. Cao D, Guo S, Allan RW et al (2009) SALL4 is a novel sensitive and specific marker of ovarian primitive germ cell tumors and is particularly useful in distinguishing yolk sac tumor from clear cell carcinoma. Am J Surg Pathol 33:894–904
6. Gokden N, Gokden M, Phan DC et al (2008) The utility of PAX-2 in distinguishing metastatic clear cell renal cell carcinoma from its morphologic mimics: an immunohistochemical study with comparison to renal cell carcinoma marker. Am J Surg Pathol 32:1462–1467
7. Lee KR, Young RH (2003) The distinction between primary and metastatic mucinous carcinomas of the ovary: gross and histologic findings in 50 cases. Am J Surg Pathol 27:281–292

MIX
Papier aus verantwortungsvollen Quellen
Paper from responsible sources
FSC® C105338

If you have any concerns about our products,
you can contact us on
ProductSafety@springernature.com

In case Publisher is established outside the EU,
the EU authorized representative is:
Springer Nature Customer Service Center GmbH
Europaplatz 3, 69115 Heidelberg, Germany

Printed by Libri Plureos GmbH
in Hamburg, Germany